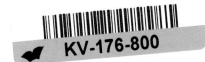
FUNDING HEALTH CARE: 2008 AND BEYOND

Report from the Leeds Castle summit

John Appleby (editor)

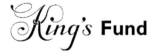

King's Fund

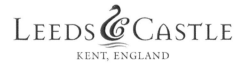

LEEDS & CASTLE

KENT, ENGLAND

The King's Fund is grateful to the trustees of the Leeds Castle Foundation for their generosity in making this summit possible.

First published 2006 by the King's Fund

Charity registration number: 207401

British Library Cataloguing in Publishing Data
A catalogue record for this publication is available from the British Library

ISBN-10: 1 85717 553 0
ISBN-13: 978 1 85717 553 0

Available from:
King's Fund
11–13 Cavendish Square
London W1G 0AN
Tel: 020 7307 2591
Fax: 020 7307 2801
Email: publications@kingsfund.org.uk
www.kingsfund.org.uk/publications

Edited by Rod Cuff
Typeset by Florence Production Ltd, Stoodleigh, Devon
Printed in the UK by the King's Fund

Contents

List of figures and tables

**Targets, targets, targets: Prospects for successful implementation
of current NHS reforms**
Mike Farrar

About the authors

Alan Maynard is Professor of Health Economics at the University of York and Chair of the York NHS Hospitals Trust. He taught economics at the University of Exeter and York before he was appointed Founding Director of the Graduate Programme in Health Economics at York. In 1983 he was appointed Founding Director of the Centre for Health Economics (CHE), and in 1996 created the York Health Policy Group in the Department of Health Sciences in York. He is also Adjunct Professor at the Centre for Health Economics Research and Evaluation at the Technology University of Sydney, Australia. He has worked as a consultant for the World Bank, the World Health Organisation and the European Commission in countries such as China, Malawi and Bolivia. During his career as an academic he has been closely involved in NHS management and policy-making.

Robert Chote was appointed Director of the Institute for Fiscal Studies in October 2002. He was formerly an adviser and speechwriter to the First Deputy Managing Director of the International Monetary Fund, working first for Stanley Fischer and then for Anne Krueger. Between 1995 and 1999, he was Economics Editor of the *Financial Times*. Previously, he served as Economics Correspondent of the *Independent* and a columnist on the *Independent on Sunday*. He is a Governor of the National Institute of Economic and Social Research and served as a member of the Statistics Advisory Committee of the Office for National Statistics. He has carried out consultancy work for organisations including the United Nations and Commonwealth Secretariat.

John Appleby is Chief Economist at the King's Fund. John has researched and published widely on many aspects of health service funding, rationing, resource allocation and performance. He previously worked as an economist with the NHS in Birmingham and London, and at the universities of Birmingham and East Anglia as Senior Lecturer in health economics. He is a visiting professor at the department of economics at City University. John's current work includes research into the impact of patient choice and payment by results. He is also acting as an adviser to the Northern Ireland Department of Finance and Personnel in respect of the implementation of his recommendations following a review of health and social care services in Northern Ireland.

Andy McKeon is Managing Director of Health at the Audit Commission. Andy was the Director of Policy at the Department of Health. During his time at the Department he was also head of primary care, and played a central role in the development of a number of White Papers.

Mike Farrar CBE is Chief Executive of West Yorkshire Strategic Health Authority. Before taking up this post in 2005, he was Chief Executive of South Yorkshire Strategic Health Authority, the first health economy in England in which all hospital trusts were awarded foundation trust status. Previously Head of Primary Care at the Department of Health, Mike led the development of primary care policy for the NHS Plan. He was the national Director of NHS Live, a programme designed to drive forward improvement and innovation in the NHS. A former semi-professional footballer, Mike was last year appointed a non-executive director of Sport England.

Executive summary

In order to help inform the debate about funding health over the next five to ten years, the King's Fund organised a meeting of senior NHS managers, Department of Health officials, Prime Ministerial policy advisers and academic health economists. It set out to consider not just the immediate question of what level of public funding is feasible and desirable during the period of next year's Comprehensive Spending Review (CSR) and beyond, but also the *process* by which such decisions should be reached and the *framework* that ought to guide and inform policy-makers. A list of participants appears at the end of this report.

As ever, the CSR will have to consider difficult spending trade-offs, but it seemed likely that the NHS could expect, as over the past seven years, to enjoy one of the larger settlements in the CSR. However, compared with past increases this could mean reduced real annual growth of between 3 per cent (roughly the long-term average trend for the NHS) and 4.4 per cent (the broad Wanless recommendation for the next CSR period under his so-called 'fully engaged' scenario).

Following presentations on key aspects of current system reforms in the NHS – including their delivery over the next few years, international comparisons, the economic background to the next CSR, possibilities for productivity improvements, the need to find rational ways to limit health care spending growth, and the current and medium-term financial situation in the NHS – a wide-ranging discussion focused on five important issues.

1: Measure what counts – health

The benefits of including routine measurement of health status as part of patients' medical records are potentially enormous – from improved measures of productivity and comparative performance benchmarking, through to the sort of information patients and purchasers need to inform their treatment and purchasing decisions.

There is no reason to delay carrying out large-scale trials to explore the potential for realising these benefits and the costs of doing so.

2: Reduce variations in performance and clinical practice

It has been evident for many years that there are largely unexplained variations in referral and operation rates, treatment thresholds, prescribing rates, primary care trusts' (PCTs') spending decisions and performance in general. Failure to tackle unnecessary variations effectively has had an adverse impact on equity as well as on efficiency.

High-impact performance variations should be identified and incentive systems designed specifically to reduce them to acceptable limits. PCTs need to justify their spending priorities explicitly, through a relationship between spending and outcomes, and trusts need to reduce variations in clinical practice beyond those related to variations in need.

3: Improve productivity

As the growth in NHS funding slows from 2008, but with demand and public expectations likely to increase, getting more benefit from every pound spent on health care will become an urgent priority.

Targets and incentive systems to improve productivity should focus on clinical quality and health as the 'product'. The reimbursement system, Payment by Results (PbR), should play a part in encouraging a more automatic mechanism to encourage the NHS to seek out more productive ways of meeting patients' health care needs.

4: Design effective incentive systems

Professionalism and vocation need to be supported and enhanced by incentive systems based on a proper understanding of the intrinsic motivations of NHS staff.

Clinical contracts and the contractual arrangements between purchasers and providers need to be reviewed in order to reward improvements in health and productivity – not just those in time and activity. Organisational incentives – such as PbR – must be ready to adapt when their real, as opposed to theoretical, impact emerges.

5: Engage clinicians

In a labour-intensive industry, doctors, nurses and other health care professionals are *the* key resource – not just clinically, but managerially too.

Greater efforts should be made to involve clinicians in the management of the NHS – through responsibility for devolved budgets and involvement and ownership of strategic management decisions.

Introduction and overview

The government has announced that there will be a second Comprehensive Spending Review (CSR) (the first one was launched in June 1997). The new review will cover the years 2008/9 to 2010/11 and will take 'a zero-based approach' to assessing the effectiveness of government departments in delivering the outputs to which they are committed.

It will also examine long-term trends and challenges that will shape public services in the next decade and it will look at how public expenditure can deliver greater efficiency and long-term investment to meet these challenges.

The CSR for the whole of government expenditure follows a period of unprecedented growth in spending on the National Health Service in the UK, which has been growing at around 7.4 per cent in real terms since 2002.

There is an expectation that these levels of growth will not be sustained beyond 2008, partly because there is a view in government that such high levels were justified for a short period to bring UK health care up to the levels of our European counterparts, and partly because the national economic outlook may demand constraints on the whole of the public sector.

The current high spending levels were underpinned by the Prime Minister's commitment in 2000 to reach the average level for the European Union and by a report from Sir Derek Wanless, who was commissioned to undertake a review of the long-term trends affecting the health service in the UK.

His report argued that the UK had fallen behind other countries in health outcomes, in part because the UK had spent less but also because it had not spent well. It concluded that the UK should devote a significantly larger share of its national income to health care over the following 20 years – reaching between 10.6 and 11.1 per cent of Gross Domestic Product (GDP) by 2022/3, up from 7.7 per cent in 2002/3.

It suggested that growth in spending should be highest in the early years, in order to allow the service to 'catch up' with other countries – the report assumed that growth in the later years would be lower.

The 2007 CSR provides the first major opportunity to revisit the funding of health since the Wanless Report and since the government embarked on its unprecedented investment in the National Health Service.

Genesis and aims of the summit

In order to help inform the debate about funding health over the next five to ten years, the King's Fund organised a meeting of senior NHS managers, Department of Health officials, Prime Ministerial policy advisers and academic health economists. It set out to consider not just the immediate question of what level of public funding is feasible and desirable during the period of the CSR and beyond, but also the *process* by which such decisions should be reached and the *framework* that ought to guide and inform policy-makers. A list of participants appears at the end of this report.

Presentations and debate at the meeting assumed that the NHS will continue to be funded from general taxation and that the current government will wish to maintain a comprehensive service free at the point of delivery.

The aim of the meeting was to provide a clear view of the options for funding health care in the immediate and medium term, building on and taking forward recent work undertaken by Sir Derek Wanless and others, including the Fund's Chief Economist, Professor John Appleby.

Challenges for system reform and financial management

Two aspects of the context to the Leeds Castle discussions need to be noted. The first is the programme of evolutionary reform of the NHS the government set in train around 2000. The second important aspect of the context – particularly over the next few years – is the need for the NHS to recover its financial position. In 2005/6 the NHS in England incurred a net deficit of £512 million, a comparatively small fraction of its total spend, but occurring at a time of unprecedented growth in funding.

The need to improve performance has driven the government's reforms of the system – from the evolving design and scope of regulators such as the Healthcare Commission and Monitor to the redesign of reimbursement systems at organisational and individual levels and the promotion of greater choice for patients.

More broadly these reforms aim to meet a clear and obvious aspiration for the NHS: that it should be a service that is patient-led, promoting health and delivering safe, high-quality care in a cost-effective way. There have been profound challenges for all aspects of the service – policy, management, clinical practice and behaviour – in meeting these goals. The reforms also have to cope with the external pressures on the NHS from increased demands and costs, and with changes in the scope of what should be considered legitimate aspects of health care.

While the reforms – in particular the focused efforts to reduce waiting times – have notched up successes, it could be argued that much more could and needs to be done to improve patients' experience of care, clinical safety and health outcomes in general. For example, patient choice is so far fairly limited and there is scope to extend it into areas which patients may find more valuable such as a much more informed choice of treatment.

There also remain persistent variations across the NHS, in the utilisation of and access to services and the sustainability of current configurations of services, but also in spending patterns and productivity and in the efficiency with which resources are used.

In the long term there are reasons to be optimistic about the sustainability of the NHS. A rising share of GDP on health care of around 3–5 per cent is easily accommodated in a growing economy, and there is evidence both here and abroad that value for money and effectiveness can be improved through service redesign and 'doing the right thing better'. Nevertheless, the recent history of reform so far suggests that there will be a need for flexibility and no shortage of difficult policy choices: Should clinicians have accountability for care and budgets along care pathways? What is the right combination of capitation and tariff to incentivise major improvements in the management of chronic diseases? Should quality and safety criteria be put against the tariff? Clearly, the policy agenda is not going to run dry quite yet.

In the short term, however, regaining financial stability for the NHS is a clear imperative. The net overspend in 2005/6 attracted many media headlines, but the service had not moved from relative financial calm to 'crisis' overnight. Taking out the effects of the system of resource accounting and budgeting, it is clear that there had been a more or less continuous deterioration in the deficit from 2000/1. Of course, in its history the NHS has previously recorded deficits but then recovered its position over a few years; it has also had years of surpluses, for which it has also been criticised. One difference now is the fact that since 1999/2000, additional annual funding has been running at more than twice the long-term rate; with more money than ever, how could the NHS overspend?

The answer is not straightforward. Part of the explanation is likely to have been a degree of miscalculation between the allocations to the NHS and the cost pressures and policy imperatives it eventually faced. In addition, some of the traditional financial safety valves – for example, letting waiting times grow – were, of course, explicitly no longer available.

And just as current stories of vacancy freezes and job losses are seen by some as cuts to services, the psychology around the need to maintain financial control at the same time as trumpeting the scale of extra funding going into the NHS meant perhaps that the discipline of *actively* ensuring such control was neglected. In addition, a degree of complacency – born perhaps of historical responses to previous deficits – was at play: previous forecast deficits often evaporated by the year end as efforts were made during the year to contain spending to budgets.

Again, the optimistic view of the current deficit position is that it can and will be dealt with. Certainly there is no doubt now of the need to maintain focus on the finances even, perhaps especially, in times of plenty. However, with one more year of the current largesse left, and a reduced level of growth for the next CSR round, the need to tackle not just the symptoms but also the underlying causes of the deficit is pressing.

This report

The Leeds Castle meeting was structured around three main themes, designed to move from the general to the specific, but with links throughout. The first part investigated views about the broad macroeconomic future, including an international view of future health care funding and thoughts on the process and framework in which NHS budget limits ought (perhaps) to be decided.

The second part tackled more detailed issues of concern to the CSR – the scope for future productivity gains, demand management, cost control, the impact of current policies on costs etc.

The third part examined the reality for the NHS of facing a medium-term future of low growth in funding.

This edited report is structured around these themes, using the presentations at the meetings and subsequent discussions of the issues by participants.

Summary of discussions

The impetus for the summit was the forthcoming Comprehensive Spending Review (CSR) in 2007 – the outcome of which many anticipate will mean a step down in the growth in NHS funding compared with the past seven years.

As the 2006 Budget stated, the 2007 CSR comes ten years after the last review, and groundwork for the CSR will include an examination of the key long-term trends and challenges that will shape the next decade – including demographic and socio-economic change, globalisation, climate and environmental change, global uncertainty and technological change. The Chancellor also announced the government's intention of starting a national debate to build a shared understanding of how the UK and public services need to respond to these challenges and, importantly, a 'far-reaching value for money programme to release the resources needed to address the challenges. . .' This will involve 'further development of the efficiency areas developed in the Gershon review, and a set of zero-based reviews of departments' baseline expenditure to assess its effectiveness in delivering the Government's long-term objectives'.

For the NHS, by 2008, the government's ambition of increasing the spending on health care to the average level of our European Union neighbours will have been all but achieved. This will be a significant success. But matching the financial inputs is only half the story, as the extensive debate and discussion following the presentations demonstrated.

Here, these discussions are summarised under common themes and concerns. While participants disagreed on some issues of detail, there was consensus in many areas.

Financial outlook

There was agreement with Robert Chote's analysis that concluded that the Chancellor's room for manoeuvre over public finances will be tight. The macroeconomic future, some suggested, may not be as bright as the recent past, with a possibility of reduced growth in the Gross Domestic Product (GDP). This could initiate a fundamental examination of the burden of the tax system and the share of public spending in the economy.

As ever, therefore, the CSR will have to consider difficult spending trade-offs, but it seemed likely that the NHS could expect, as over the past seven years, to enjoy one of the larger settlements in the CSR. However, compared with past increases this could mean reduced real annual growth of between 3 per cent (roughly the long-term average trend for the NHS) and 4.4 per cent (the broad Wanless recommendation for the next CSR period under his so-called 'fully engaged' scenario).

Although the headlines from the Wanless review of future NHS funding perhaps naturally focused on the financial inputs to the service and the 'catch up' recommendations, a key question was the extent to which (and over what period) the NHS would catch up in terms of its outputs and, importantly, outcomes.

There was agreement that the large financial investment in the NHS over the past seven years had produced successes – greatly reduced waiting times, for example, and increased numbers of frontline staff. However, in the midst of plenty, the fact that the NHS moved further into the red in 2005/6 did not just seem paradoxical, but appeared to support the views of long-term critics of the NHS that it was provider-dominated and inherently incapable of delivering the level and quality of care – efficiently and on budget – that the population had a right to expect.

But, as was pointed out, not only did the overspend represent less than 1 per cent of the total NHS budget, but this level of deficit was not unusual by historical standards and had, indeed, been tolerated in the past.

Clearly, however, the financial and policy environments had changed, with more money going into the NHS, a tighter accounting framework and policies such as Payment by Results (PbR) injecting a new and tougher set of incentives into the system. While the new system reforms – such as PbR – were not the root cause of deficits (Wales, for instance, incurred similar levels of deficits in 2005/6 without a similar reform agenda), they are expected (indeed, designed) to generate greater financial uncertainty for parts of the NHS in order to stimulate greater responsiveness and efficiency. They could also, however, potentially exacerbate the speed of financial distress for some organisations.

Other reasons for individual deficits included the fact that large Private Finance Initiative (PFI) schemes, mergers and turnover of board members had in some cases distracted senior management from their ongoing financial control duties.

But while deficits were a serious issue, the key question concerning the past seven years' additional investment (and one pertinent to future investment) was: what had happened to efficiency and to the quality of care? And, further, how had health improved?

Measuring returns to health care investment

While for many years a major complaint had been that the NHS was underfunded, the plaintive question now was: where has the money gone?

There are many ways to answer this, but there was strong agreement that the lack of routine measurement of health outcomes in the NHS was a major block in providing the answer to the fundamental question of how inputs were linked to outcomes.

While better information about health outcomes could also help in understanding the relationship between inputs and outcomes, and thus help inform NHS investment decisions, there was some disagreement on where the NHS might currently reside on the input–outcome 'curve', and hence the extent to which additional investment would be worthwhile. For example, while it may be the case that for elective services the NHS was near the 'flat' of the curve, it was probably not true for mental health care or stroke services. Furthermore, identifying optimal NHS spend on the basis of the health returns on investment was also problematic: stopping spending when marginal returns were zero would be too late, but at what point before this would such action be just right?

Understanding and measuring the health outcomes or benefits of spending was not just desirable at the level of the whole system, but was also essential within the NHS. In a low(er)-growth future, prioritising spending becomes more acute, and primary care trusts (PCTs), it was felt, need to justify spending patterns. With cash becoming scarcer, what were the relative (health outcome) merits of investing more heavily in primary care, for example? And would a focus on health care spending on the elderly and the poor be more likely to improve the health returns on each health care pound than would investment targeted at other groups?

It was recognised that there now seems to be some impetus within the Department of Health to explore the issue of measuring health outcomes, and that it was vital to invest in understanding what measures to use and what technical issues need to be addressed.

While measuring the health benefits produced by health *care* spending was considered vital, it was also recognised that there is plenty of evidence to show that although some health services are good investments if spending was directed into the right interventions, other *non*-health care services (such as education) have also been identified as having significant impacts on a population's health outcomes.

Further, the obverse of health outcomes from non-health care services is non-health outcomes – eg, employment and reduced benefit payments – from health care spending. The extent to which this multiple-output argument can justify higher spending on the NHS may be debatable; but, more broadly, understanding where best to make investment in order to achieve health gains was clearly important, and this involved generating quantifiable evidence about benefits.

Improving productivity

Another issue that dominated many of the discussions at the summit (and one intimately linked to the measurement of health outcomes) was productivity.

There was agreement that there was considerable scope for the NHS to improve productivity – although it was pointed out that because annual productivity increases in the rest of the economy tended to average around 2 per cent, it may be unwise to assume that the NHS could achieve more than this without adversely affecting the quality of care. Nevertheless, with abundant evidence of persistent and largely unexplained variations in performance across the NHS, there seemed to be prima facie evidence that there were productivity gains to be made. Moreover, aiming high may be the way to really engage NHS staff and to generate more innovative thinking about productivity improvements.

Although the NHS will undoubtedly face a tighter financial future, this was not thought necessarily to be a problem. Rather, when coupled with system reforms such as PbR and patient choice, it could act as an incentive to seek out productivity improvements. Key questions raised were how to diffuse such incentives throughout the system, how to ensure productivity gains were real and sustainable, and how to engage clinicians in all this.

While throwing money at a problem can be a way of solving it, a better understanding of how recent benefits had actually been achieved is required. For example, recent reductions in waiting times do not appear mainly to have been achieved from increases in activity. Improving productivity is also about improving processes and re-engineering systems to achieve gains in benefits. The relationship between inputs and outputs in health care was a complex one – and not necessarily linear: more in does not necessarily lead to more out. More thought, it was suggested, needed to be given to redistributive tactics to improve quality and productivity – but this would require a much greater understanding of the returns or benefits from different investment strategies and service areas, and a deeper understanding of persistent and largely unexplained variations in performance.

The 'elephant in the room' in many discussions about NHS productivity is, however, the nature of the 'product'. The straightforward answer is 'health', but as previous discussions emphasised, the NHS (like all health systems) fails to measure what matters most to patients.

While traditional NHS productivity measures have centred on ratios of various inputs (money, labour, beds) to various outputs (patients treated, ambulance journeys, outpatient attendances), there was a need to adjust such measures for changes in the quality of the output. It is not good enough simply to count cars rolling off the production line when the car itself has changed from a Mini to a Lexus.

It was essential to develop the right productivity metrics to reflect properly the business the NHS is in, but the question would remain of how to improve productivity. For example, how can the massive investment in information technology (IT) planned for the NHS be used to improve health outputs rather than simply (*sic*) to computerise administrative functions?

One view was that productivity improvements generally arise from the entry of new providers into an industry. If this is right, then the current system reforms of the NHS need to grapple with ways not only to facilitate this but to deal with the linked inevitability of exit too, through well-thought-out failure regimes and regulatory intervention. Such a regime would have to take a 'whole health economy' perspective in order to tackle problems where, for example, providers found themselves losing business but unable to cut their costs. The temptation on the part of the provider in these circumstances would be to trade their way out of trouble, but in so doing they may transfer their financial problem to commissioners.

Although commissioning has so far taken a back seat in recent NHS reforms, the need to support and bolster PCTs' purchasing role was now being recognised. An important part of this ought to be development of quality standards and productivity measures and for these to be built into commissioning contracts.

The history of productivity gains in the NHS was not felt to be one of sustained (and sustainable) improvement. Traditional top-down productivity and efficiency-improvement tactics – characterised by the 'take the money away first and ask the productivity questions later' approach – may produce short-term gains, but were thought to be inappropriate in the longer term. There was agreement that NHS organisations and NHS staff had to internalise the need to improve productivity. It was also felt to be absolutely crucial to engage clinical staff in this – for example, through devolution of budgets, real involvement in managerial decisions, the development of strategy, the design of care pathways and so on.

Better incentives to 'do the right thing'

A common thread that ran throughout all the discussions was how to incentivise not just NHS organisations and staff to 'do the right thing' – improve productivity, maximise take-up of innovative service delivery, provide the right care at the right time to the right patients – but also patients and the public.

It was essential to get the right productivity measures, health outcome metrics and process information in place; but the next steps were about deciding how to deal with this information and what incentive mechanisms would be most effective in producing the right responses.

Although current system reforms – in particular PbR and patient choice – in theory introduce some strong rewards and sanctions, underpinning these changes are assumptions about what will motivate NHS organisations, staff and patients. Do providers want to maximise income? What factors will drive patients' choices? What are the potential adverse trade-offs between financial and non-financial incentives?

Clearly, the current system reforms represent something of an experiment, and it was suggested that there was a case for piloting more and rolling out less. However, it was recognised that there were limits to testing new policies, and that it could always be argued that more evidence could be gathered before policy was formulated and implemented. It was noted, however, that there was certainly room for better modelling of how the systems as a whole would develop and change because of changes being introduced and to test for risks and the probabilities of expected outcomes.

There was agreement that, unless the motivations of all the actors in the system are understood, it is difficult to design effective incentive systems that not only prompt action and maximise the 'correct' response, but minimise perverse reactions.

Even where motivations are thought to be well understood, it is still difficult to get the incentive system right first time. What was also required was experimentation with incentives. For example, how can PbR be adapted in order to encourage greater delivery of cost-effective care? And could a similar tariff system deliver improvements in primary care? How were the incentives embodied in PbR to be transmitted to the frontline and diffused throughout hospitals? To what extent should the incentives being faced by organisations be made to 'bite' on individuals and teams within organisations?

On this, some scepticism was expressed about whether current reforms – in particular, changes in contracts for clinicians – had produced much positive behavioural change. As with PbR, it was thought that more experimentation was needed to explore the sort of incentives that could be used at the level of individual staff – such as fee for service or the use of health outcome targets in clinical contracts.

While there has been considerable focus on incentivising the supply side in the NHS, it was also argued that incentives need to be considered for the demand side too – commissioning and patient choice. With the right sort of performance information on quality of care and health outcomes, commissioners and patients could become more active in the system, helping to drive up quality through their respective decisions on purchasing and choice.

Dealing with demand

While the phrase 'demand management' had rather pejorative connotations – suggestive of restrictions on individuals' rights to access care – all health care systems, no matter how they were funded, had to use one mechanism (for example, prices) or another (such as waiting lists) to achieve equilibrium.

The need for equitable (and ethically acceptable) ways of ensuring long-term sustainable equilibrium between demand and supply in a system that has rejected price as the key factor for allocating resources is, of course, not new. However, in the light of current and future circumstances it was felt that greater urgency was required to understand and then to manage demand pressures in the system.

In the short term, dealing with deficits means finding ways to limit expenditure – through productivity increases or by acting to curtail demand (although probably by combining both approaches). One example where demand has been increasing at a substantial rate was the nearly 30 per cent rise in emergency admissions between 1998 and 2004 (compared with a 5 per cent increase in elective admissions). Incentives imposed via the 2006/7 PbR tariffs (that is, reducing the tariff for increases in emergency admissions over a certain limit) should incentivise hospitals to seek ways to limit demand in this part of the system. However, the impact of this might be attenuated if the cause of rising emergency admissions was beyond the control of providers. There was also a danger that health outcomes could be adversely affected by a simple focus on, for example, reducing hospital referrals.

Looking to the medium term, questions were raised about the fuelling of demand – in part as a result of the success of the NHS in reducing waiting times (would patient expectations simply rise to demand even shorter waits?) and in part through policies such as patient choice. Some argued, for example, that patient choice may be a costly policy to pursue, given the need for trusts to hold extra capacity. Further, it might be that the benefits to patients of the actual choice on offer (that is, a choice of institution) may be minimal, because what patients really wanted to be able to choose was the detail of their care – including the clinician or team.

Nevertheless, it was argued that survey evidence indicated not only that people were pro-choice when in need of care but that the less well-off were more pro-choice than others. In addition, rather than limiting choice, there may be a case for extending it in other directions – for example, to a choice of commissioner. It was noted that such a move was not on the current NHS reform agenda and that it would limit the development of population-based health care on a regional basis.

In relation to demand management and the involvement of patients, others argued that patients' expert programmes demonstrated that, when patients were more informed and involved in their own care, their choices and decisions often led to better treatment compliance, medication was reduced and use of secondary care was also reduced. Knowing more and being more active does not necessarily lead to increased demand.

Given the knowledge that supply influences demand in health care, it was suggested that the NHS could in part manage demand by managing supply. Supply-induced and supplier-induced demand needed to be better understood, however, in order to identify how and where supply and supplier decisions could be influenced to better manage demand. For example, more narrowly defining what the NHS should provide could be self-defeating; excluding health promotion activities, for example, could simply lead to greater use of other NHS services.

Moving forward: lessons for the future

For many in the NHS, grappling with the implementation of system-wide reforms such as Payment by Results, choice, further organisational restructuring and – of course – the need to regain financial control, these are turbulent times; but in many ways it was ever thus. The medium-term financial future for the NHS will be less generous than the recent past, and is likely to feel even tighter. However, as the summary of discussions above indicates, emerging from all this are some key issues that the NHS and policy-makers need to engage with.

1: Measure what counts – health

The benefits of including routine measurement of health status as part of patients' medical records are potentially enormous – from improved measures of productivity and comparative performance benchmarking, through to the sort of information patients and purchasers need to inform their treatment and purchasing decisions.

There is no reason to delay carrying out large-scale trials to explore the potential for realising these benefits and the costs of doing so.

2: Reduce variations in performance and clinical practice

It has been evident for many years that there are largely unexplained variations in referral and operation rates, treatment thresholds, prescribing rates, primary care trusts' (PCTs') spending decisions and performance in general. Failure to tackle unnecessary variations effectively has had an adverse impact on equity as well as on efficiency.

High-impact performance variations should be identified and incentive systems designed specifically to encourage their reduction to acceptable limits. PCTs need to justify their spending priorities explicitly, through a relationship between spending and outcomes, and trusts need to reduce variations in clinical practice beyond those related to variations in need.

3: Improve productivity

As the growth in NHS funding slows from 2008, but with demand and public expectations likely to increase, getting more benefit from every health care pound will become an urgent priority.

Targets and incentive systems to improve productivity should focus on clinical quality and health as the 'product'. The reimbursement system, Payment by Results, should play a part in encouraging a more automatic mechanism to encourage the NHS to seek out more productive ways of meeting patients' health care needs.

4: Design effective incentive systems

Professionalism and vocation need to be supported and enhanced by incentive systems based on a proper understanding of the intrinsic motivations of NHS staff.

Clinical contracts and the contractual arrangements between purchasers and providers need to be reviewed in order to reward improvements in health and productivity – not just those in time and activity. Organisational incentives – such as Payment by Results – must be ready to adapt when their real, as opposed to theoretical, impact emerges.

5: Engage clinicians

In a labour-intensive industry, doctors, nurses and other health care professionals are *the* key resource – not just clinically, but managerially too.

Greater efforts should be made to involve clinicians in the management of the NHS – through responsibility for devolved budgets and involvement and ownership of strategic management decisions.

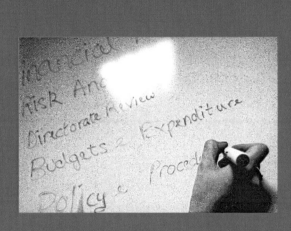

Part 1

Macroeconomic background, international trends and spending-decision frameworks

Key questions

- What can international health care spending trends tell us?
- What are the medium-term prospects for the UK economy, taxation and public spending?
- Is there a more rational/evidence-based process that can be used to set global health care budgets?

'Keeping up with the Joneses'
International trends in health care spending

Alan Maynard

'Keeping up with the Joneses'
International trends in health care spending

Alan Maynard[1]

'Keeping up with the Joneses is a popular phrase in many parts of the English-speaking world referring to the common desire to be seen to be as good as one's neighbours or contemporaries, thus maintaining a favourable image in comparison with them. To fail to 'keep up with the Joneses' is perceived as demonstrating one's socio-economic or cultural inferiority.'
(Wikipedia.org)

Introduction

The Labour government inherited a relatively frugally funded National Health Service (NHS) in 1997 that was observably inefficient in its use of resources, as evidenced, for example, in considerable unexplained variations in clinical practice in hospitals (for example, Yates 1995), a practically data-free primary care system that politicians described as the 'best in the world' (Bloor, Maynard and Street 2000) and an evidence base and administrative data systems (eg, Hospital Episode Statistics [HES]) that were not routinely used in clinical practice and management. Its response to these efficiency and funding challenges was to indulge in an evidence-free 'redisorganisation' of the structure of the NHS, including the creation of primary care trusts (PCTs) and the abolition of GP fundholding and trust hospitals. These changes were complemented by investments in 'quality', in particularly the National Service Frameworks (NSFs), and in regulation, in particular the National Institute for Health and Clinical Excellence (NICE) and the Commission for Health Improvement (CHI).

However, these changes did little to resolve the main political issue associated with the NHS: waiting time for elective care. In a Damascene-like conversion, initiated it is said by the Chancellor, Gordon Brown, and taken up with enthusiasm by Tony Blair, the government chose to mitigate this along with associated 'ills' of the NHS (for example, alleged capacity shortfalls and maintenance backlogs) with an ambitious investment programme aimed at keeping up with the European Joneses by shifting United Kingdom (UK) expenditure to the European Union (EU) average. This is being implemented by large annual increases in funding and by 'continuous revolution' in policies aimed at creating uncertainty and change in work practices. Unfortunately, despite the inherent merits of

---

1 The author would like to acknowledge the help of Dr Karen Bloor in preparing this paper.

some of these policies in creating contestability and incentivising change, they lack a coherent strategic framework and a regulatory structure to ensure expenditure control, improved efficiency and greater equity in the distribution of health care, let alone to ensure health.

What can be learned from the international Joneses about the ends and the means used in this bold, expensive and largely unevaluated social experiment?

International trends

The principal driver of health care expenditure is the rate of growth of Gross Domestic Product (GDP). In the past ten years the growth rates of the component parts of the European Monetary Union countries (in particular Germany, France, Italy and Spain) have been low, while the British economy has grown modestly but steadily. This success has enabled the government to fund the Blair bonanza for the NHS and drive the UK share of GDP spent on the NHS to the European average – that is, a target of around 9 per cent as opposed to about 6.5 per cent in 2000.

Data from the Organisation for Economic Co-operation and Development (OECD) for health care expenditure in US dollars, adjusted for purchasing power (*see* Figure 1 below), show that over the decade to 2002 (the latest date for which there is consistent cross-country data) countries such as Australia, Canada, Germany, France, the Netherlands, Sweden and the UK experienced gradual increases in spending in the range $2000 to $3000 per capita, with the UK spending least in this group The US remains an outlier, with per capita expenditure in excess of $5000 and high annual rates of inflation, currently around 10 per cent for insurance premiums, with 16 per cent of GDP spent on fragmented, inefficient and inequitable systems of care.

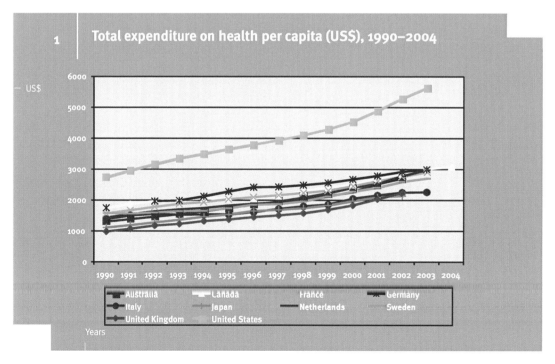

Source: OECD health data 2005

OECD data for the public–private mix in the decade to 2002 (*see* Figure 2 below) shows little change except in the Netherlands. In each of these countries except the USA, the role of the state was and is dominant. Even in the USA, government expenditure is 40 per cent of the total (one paper has re-estimated this to be 60 per cent). Only in the Netherlands does there appear to have been a significant increase in the role of the private sector.

Comparative data also show that staffing levels for doctors and nurses were relatively static (*see* Figures 3 and 4 overleaf), with the UK having the lowest levels of doctors of around 2 per thousand population, compared with levels near or above 3 for the other countries. Hospital bed stocks (*see* Figure 5, p 21) generally declined over the period, with Japan an extraordinarily high outlier and the UK at the bottom of this distribution.

Thus the UK spent less than other OECD countries and had lower levels of doctor, nurses and hospital bed stocks. What health did these varying levels of input and associated processes of care produce? The measurement of 'success' in health care systems in terms of improving patients' physical and mental well-being is generally very poor, with policy-makers inferring in an evidence-free manner that if you put more resources in, you get more health out. Life expectancy generally increased in the decade to 2002 (*see* Figure 6, p 21), with the Japanese being the best performers and the UK near the bottom of the pack. The incomplete data on self-perceived health status (*see* Figure 7, p 22) show little improvement over time, with Japan apparently performing badly. Obviously, life expectancy and perceived health status may be affected by many inputs other than health.

Where to now with NHS expenditure?

The waiting-time imperatives, along with international comparisons, apparently convinced the government to increase NHS expenditure sharply in the period to 2008. Owing to an

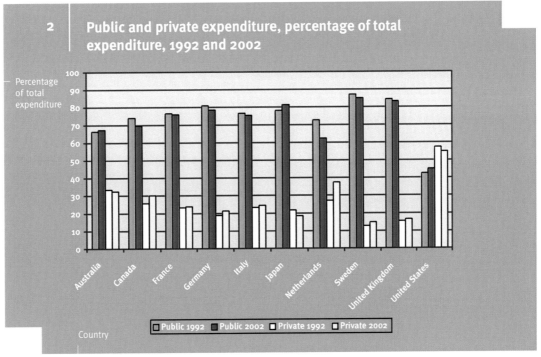

2 | **Public and private expenditure, percentage of total expenditure, 1992 and 2002**

Source: OECD health data 2005

unusual period of modest but sustained growth in GDP, the government has been able to adhere to these promises. However, at the same time it has adopted a bewildering array of new policies to create 'constructive discomfort' (Stevens 2004). Some of these, for instance Payment by Results (PbR), have created incentives to increase activity but, like the doctors' pay awards, have created no incentive to measure and manage clinical activity systematically in order to produce greater efficiency.

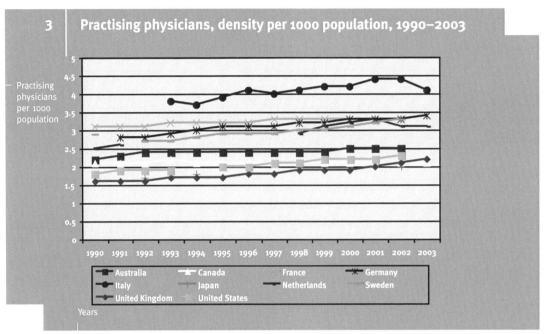

Source: OECD health data 2005

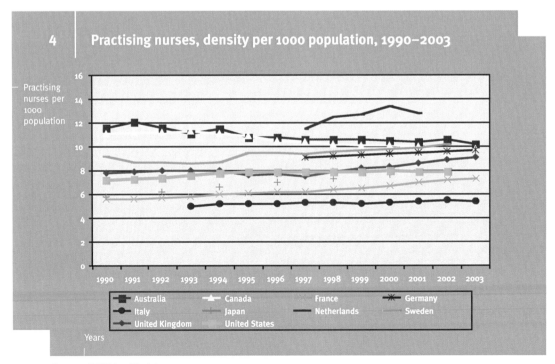

Source: OECD health data 2005

Not only have crucial areas of activity been left unmanaged, but some of the policies appear to be in conflict. For instance, PbR induces greater activity and consequent financial pressure, which pushes some PCTs over their weighted capitation-budget allocation targets. PCTs can play 'pass the parcel bomb' with such deficits, but this does not resolve the problem of using effective incentive devices such as PbR within a

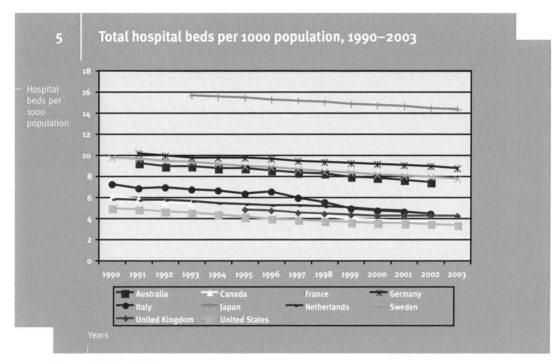

Source: OECD health data 2005

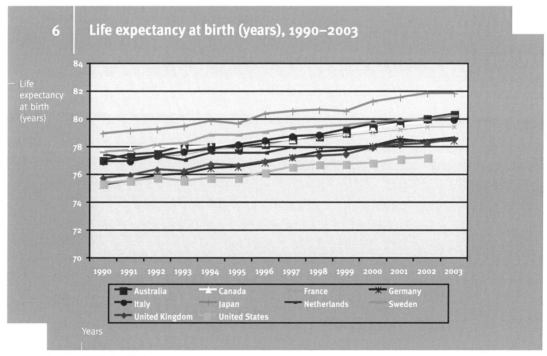

Source: OECD health data 2005

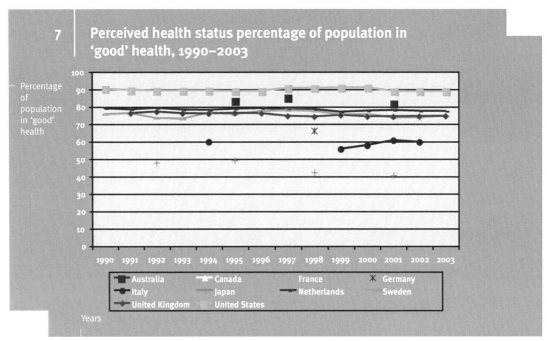

7 Perceived health status percentage of population in 'good' health, 1990–2003

Percentage of population in 'good' health

Legend: Australia, Canada, France, Germany, Italy, Japan, Netherlands, Sweden, United Kingdom, United States

Years

Source: OECD health data 2005

cash-limited system that has clear equity targets of the 'Resources Allocation Working Party' (RAWP) type. Furthermore, much of this policy-making appears to have ignored the evidence base; for example, whether you look at the US, Germany, South Korea or Taiwan, tariffs of the Diagnostic Related Group (DRG) type increase activity. They can also lead to the restructuring of the hospital system, as in the USA in the 1980s and in Germany currently with the increased sale of municipal hospitals to the private sector. This evidence base could have been used to produce a better-informed NHS policy: in particular an improved regulatory structure to manage the reform of the hospital sector, for example by setting and enforcing rules for market entry, exit and merger for public and private providers.

The pertinent issue now is whether the uncertainty created by the continuous and usually evidence-free reforms of NHS structures and processes is constructive or destructive. The inflationary shocks of doctors' pay awards; NICE appraisals that rarely say no to new technologies and ignore the scope for the removal of inefficient old technologies; public expectations of even shorter waiting times and further 'quality improvements', sometimes in areas of marginal cost-effectiveness such as cancer care; all these have created a dynamic that is costly and may absorb most of the new annual growth money (Appleby 2006).

The Treasury's position is associated with their late awareness of the problems of the current reforms. In material used by the *Financial Times* in January (Timmins 2006), it is clear that they are now aware of the cost and relative lack of quid pro quo in the doctors' pay awards (predicted years ago by some, eg, Maynard and Sheldon 2002; Maynard and Bloor 2003), which has created the best-paid practitioners in Europe. The Treasury has also become aware of the relatively high price of drugs in the UK, now likely to be challenged by the Office of Fair Trading review of the Pharmaceutical Price Regulation Scheme (Office of Fair Trading 2006).

The capacity of the UK economy to fund continuing high levels of growth in NHS expenditure is constrained by the rate of growth of the economy and the size of the public sector. The former is likely to be modest – 2 to 3 per cent per annum at best in the years after 2008 – and the latter is constrained by the politics and rhetoric around the size of the public sector. With rhetoric favouring the 'superiority' of private-sector activity, despite the lessons of Enron, Equitable Life and Marconi, it remains politically difficult for government to increase the size of the public sector. Thus, politics and economic growth forecasts will probably restrict NHS annual expenditure growth to 3 per cent from 2008. If the NHS is prioritised beyond this growth path, other public services, some of which may produce improvements in population health more cost effectively, will be cut back.

A modest growth rate for NHS funding will create substantial challenges. The combined forces of an ageing population and technological 'creep' could be managed if rationing were explicit and the criterion of relative cost-effectiveness were to be implemented by a 'nastier' NICE. This would require political robustness typically absent around these issues, as it is around system restructuring, in particular hospital closures. However, the associated inflationary pressure from public expectations and incentive systems created by PbR will be more difficult to manage. The pharmaceutical industry, for example, produces drugs of marginal cost-effectiveness but markets them through the media and patient lobby groups in ways that deny the fact that life is finite and death certain. Again this is epitomised by the extraordinary success of cancer-related lobbies. Countervailing 'academic marketing' based on the evidence as seen in the Cochrane Collaboration database remains weak, thereby increasing pressure on government to spend more.

What are the lessons from international experience?

The lessons from international experience and from the evidence base are clear and strong, but generally ignored by policy-makers anxious to reinvent the wheel and 'surprisingly' discover costs and benefits similar to those in policies used worldwide. International evidence and experience has generated ten laws of health economics:

1. On the demand side of the NHS policy debate, there is a cycle of advocacy proposing alternative funding sources as a solution to ill-defined system problems. The **first law of health economics** is that expenditure equals income (*see* Figure 8 overleaf). Those who advocate increased NHS expenditure may often be the beneficiaries of it in terms of career enhancement and increased remuneration. Therefore it is not unusual to see provider groups such as doctors and drug companies advocating increased expenditure, which may increase their incomes. The consequence of the first law is that it is essential to inspect the motivation of those advocating more expenditure, to determine whether it is merely income-enhancing or to what extent it increases population health.

2. The **second law of health economics** is that advocates of changes in NHS funding may be seeking to redistribute the burden of financing health care provision, usually from the more affluent to the poor. Thus advocacy of the replacement of some part of tax finance with user charges should be seen for what it is:

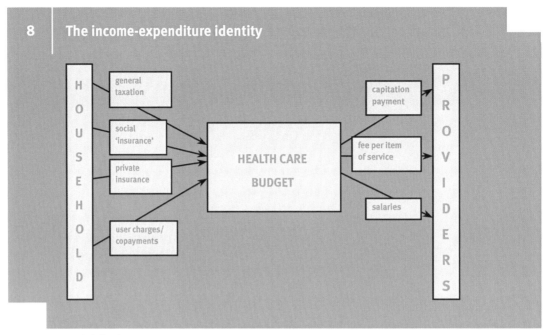

Source: Reinhardt 1984

In the present structure of health care delivery, most proposals for 'patient participation in health care financing' reduce to misguided or cynical efforts to tax the ill and/or drive up the total cost of health care while shifting some of the burden out of government budgets.
(Stoddart, Barer and Evans 1994)

Advocacy of private for-profit insurance, usually with tax subsidies as in Australia, is likely to create cost inflation, greater inequity and no efficiency gain (Hall and Maynard 2005). The Australian policy reforms, while wholly consistent with the ideological goals of the Howard government, have driven up private insurance coverage from 30 to 45 per cent, with subsidies to the relatively affluent costing over $2 billion annually. Furthermore, as insurance premiums usually inflate by a multiple of two or three times the general rate of inflation, the tax revenue loss from such subsidies grows very rapidly. Such policies inflate provider incomes but do not produce cost-effective health improvements, because insurers are generally poor price-makers and managers of clinical practice.

The adoption of social insurance typically reduces the redistributive impact of tax-based funding systems. Thus, the government's decision to use National Insurance rather than income tax to fund the Blair reforms produced less redistribution from the affluent to the poor. So a consequence of the second law of health economics is to warn against the advocates of changes in NHS funding, because they generally wish to shift funding burdens from the more affluent and healthy to the ill, who tend to be poor and elderly.

3. The **third law of health economics** suggests that expenditure control is best achieved by predominantly tax-funded and cash-limited health care systems. The evidence to support this can be seen in the expenditure histories of the UK, Scandinavian and New Zealand health care systems. The third law implies that 'single pipe' tax-funded and cash-

limited funding arrangements form a necessary condition for expenditure control. Political largesse during election cycles may ensure that the sufficient conditions for expenditure control are not always met in such systems.

4. The first three laws may give expenditure control and some equity in the distribution of funding burdens, but they guarantee neither efficiency in the supply of health care nor equity in the distribution of health care and health. The **fourth law of health economics** is that supply creates its own demand. Consumers are not generally the best judges of the efficiency of alternative diagnostic and therapeutic interventions, and typically delegate choices to their agents, the doctors. This gives providers the capacity to generate unnecessary (ie, cost-ineffective) demand, which may also enhance their income and status but do little to enhance the health status of the population.

5. The **fifth law of health economics** is that greater spending reveals unmet demand in an increasingly medicalised society. This is nicely epitomised by the problems created by increasing diagnostic capacity. In some areas (eg, Alberta in Canada) there is evidence that increased investment in diagnostic capacity increases waiting times, as the 'hidden iceberg of illness' that is thereby revealed increases pressure on diagnostic and treatment capacity. This is clearly an issue for the NHS and for the 18-week waiting-time target, where driving up, for instance, magnetic resonance imaging rates from 20 to 35 per 1000 will increase pressure on resources. The potential for a vicious circle whereby more investment creates more frustration with service delivery is also evidenced by continental Europe, where higher expenditure is accompanied by dissatisfaction with services (Dixon and Mossialos 2002).

6. The **sixth law of health economics** is that increased investment will only produce health gains if it is targeted at those interventions that are of proven cost-effectiveness. Ideally, priorities should have been set across all the National Service Frameworks, waiting-time initiatives, NICE guidance and the plethora of other government 'priorities'. Without this, resource allocation is segmented and prey to the non-evidence-based advocacy of patient and provider groups.

7. Even if this was done, not all health care demand could be met. The **seventh law of health economics** is that the rationing of health care is unavoidable. Rationing involves depriving patients of care from which they would benefit and which they would like to consume (Williams 1998). Rationing is politically difficult but ubiquitous; it is unavoidable and has to be based on cost-effectiveness and humane caring at the end of life.

8. Rationing is made more difficult by the **eighth law of health economics:** that even if priorities are pursued efficiently on the basis of relative cost-effectiveness, there are severe capacity constraints. As predicted (Maynard and Sheldon 2002), these capacity constraints create rents for provider groups, whereby additional funding is absorbed in higher pay with little effect on activity volume or quality. Policies to increase labour supply in the short term, such as overseas recruitment, private contracting and non-evidence-based changes in the skill mix (Lankshear *et al* 2005), may be inflationary in the medium term when applied in conjunction with the output of a 50 per cent increase in medical-school intake in the past six years, because many practitioners demand 'suitable' employment in the medium term.

9. The **ninth law of health economics** is that health care is not the only investment option that may increase population health. Investment in education increases earnings over the life cycle and is associated with changed behaviours that produce health, for example, less smoking. Further, investment in reducing poverty leads to changed behaviours in adults that improve not only their health but also that of their children, thereby reducing health inequalities. As Grossman has emphasised for a quarter of a century, consumers demand health, not medical care, and the policy and research challenge is to identify the inputs that create health most efficiently across a range of social policy options (Grossman 2000).

10. The **tenth law of health economics** is that incentives are ubiquitous and powerful and need to be focused, using evidence and administrative data to improve efficiency and equity. A nice example of this is the work of Dr Karen Bloor for the Department of Health. The production of activity charts showing variation and the relative performance of consultants by individual hospital (*see* Figures 9 and 10 below and opposite) posed pertinent questions that were ignored in the design of the 2004 consultant contract. Instead of demanding managerial investigation of these variations and using incentives to shift the mean of the activity distribution, the Department ignored its own data and gave a large pay increase to practitioners, with no quid pro quo for the taxpayer in terms of activity or outcome enhancement (Bloor and Maynard 2002; Maynard and Bloor 2003).

Incentivising health care activity may not improve patient outcomes. As the joke goes: 'The operation was a success but the patient died!' The remarkable reluctance of health care systems worldwide to measure outcomes has been mitigated recently by analysis of mortality rates at hospital and consultant levels. This analysis is often difficult because of

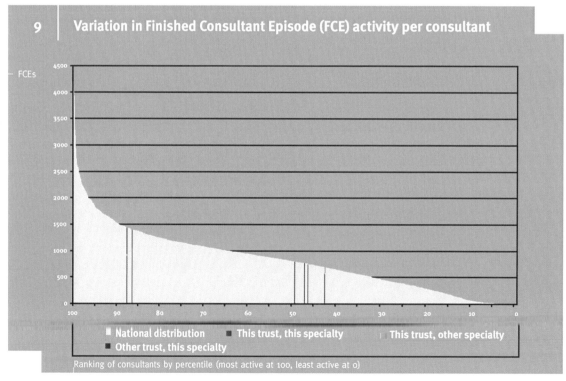

9   **Variation in Finished Consultant Episode (FCE) activity per consultant**

Ranking of consultants by percentile (most active at 100, least active at 0)

■ National distribution   ■ This trust, this specialty   ▢ This trust, other specialty
■ Other trust, this specialty

Source: Ranked activity (FCEs) per consultant in general surgery, 2001/2 data
Anonymous NHS Trust

the problems of case-mix adjustment and small numbers. However, most patients do not die in hospital, but hopefully their physical and mental functioning is improved. Is it? Why do insurer-purchasers and NHS-purchasers generally fail, with the exception of BUPA's use of patient-reported outcome measures since 1999, to measure success? Generic measures have been translated into dozens of languages and used in thousands of clinical trials, but no country has adopted them for routine use in clinical practice. (Kind and Williams 2004; Appleby and Devlin 2005).

There are many causes of this, of which the lack of incentives is a very powerful factor. Imagine a reform of the GP Quality Outcomes Framework (QOF) that paid these entrepreneurs to collect such data routinely at every patient consultation. If Practice-Based Budgeting was also properly incentivised, GPs would identify poor consultant performers and divert custom away from these providers. Furthermore, they could reduce their tariff payments for poor-quality care.

Hopefully, such long-advocated notions will be adopted as the funding pressures intensify in the NHS. They epitomise the need not only to measure activity and outcomes, using routine data that have been collected and ignored for decades (for example, Hospital Episode Statistics), but also to incentivise their use so that extraordinary and well-established practice variations are mitigated and outcome quality is assured.

So why are these laws of health economics generally ignored? Is it because of the modesty of shy, retiring health economists?! Or is it because senior policy makers are unaware of or uninterested in this evidence base? Campbell remarked nearly 40 years ago that all health care reform is social experimentation on a vulnerable population, and that

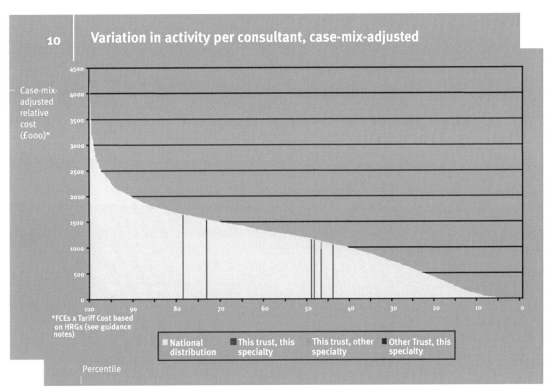

Source: Ranked activity (case-mix-adjusted*) per consultant in general surgery, 2001/2 data
Anonymous NHS Trust

for politicians there are threats to evaluating the success of this experimentation, and 'safety behind the veil of ignorance' (Campbell 1969). Sadly, the health care reform virus worldwide continues to be poorly evidence-based and rarely evaluated. Politicians and policy-makers clearly do not wish to be 'confused' by facts!

Overview

'Keeping up with the Joneses' in UK health care reform has created substantial inflationary pressures, and may improve neither the efficiency nor the equity of health care systems, let alone produce demonstrable improvements in population health. Developed and middle-income countries continue to increase health care expenditure at significant rates, but the forces driving this funding inflation, such as ageing and technological change, are moderate if they are well managed with evidence. The inflationary pressures that are less easy to control include public expectations of immortality and illness-free lives, pretensions fuelled by provider groups who are driven by self-interest to increase expenditure on marginally cost-effective therapies.

The lessons to be learned from international evidence are that there is inefficiency in the use of resources in all health care systems, with clinical practice everywhere exhibiting large unexplained and unmanaged variations in practice, with technological inflation that is often not evidence-based, and with inadequate measures 'to protect the public from harmful and useless interventions' (Chalmers 2005; Maynard 2005). The keys to creating a more efficient and equitable health care system are, first, 'hard' and modest budget increases for the NHS; and second, the incentivisation of improvements in productivity by purchasers who measure and manage providers by making use of data about activity and outcome. It really is not difficult, if only the laws of health economics could bite into the decision-making processes in Whitehall!

References

Appleby J (2006). *Where's the Money Going*? London: King's Fund.

Appleby J, Devlin N (2005). *Measuring NHS Success*. Dr Foster Ethics Committee, City University and King's Fund.

Bloor K, Maynard A (2002). 'Consultants: managing them means measuring them'. *Health Service Journal*, vol 112, 19 December, pp 10–11.

Bloor K, Maynard A, Street A (2000). 'The cornerstone of Labour's "new NHS": reforming primary care', in *Reforming Markets in Health Care*, Smith PC ed, pp 18–44. Milton Keynes: Open University Press.

Campbell DT (1969). 'Reforms as experiments', *American Psychologist*, vol 24, pp 409–29.

Chalmers I (2005). 'If evidence-informed policy works in practice, does it matter if it doesn't work in theory?' *Evidence and Theory*, vol 1, 2, pp 227–42.

Dixon A, Mossialos E (eds) (2002). *Healthcare Systems in Eight Countries: Trends and challenges*. Commissioned by the Health Trends Group (the Wanless report group), London: HM Treasury.

Grossman M (2000). 'The human capital model', in *Handbook of Health Economics, volume 1A*, Culyer AJ and Newhouse JP eds, pp 347–408. Amsterdam: North Holland.

Hall J, Maynard A (2005). 'Healthcare lessons from Australia: what can Michael Howard learn from John Howard?' *British Medical Journal*, vol 350, pp 357–59.

Kind P, Williams A (2004). 'Measuring success in health care: the time has come to do it properly!' *Health Policy Matters*. 9 March. Available online at: www.york.ac.uk/depts/hstd/pubs/hpmindex.htm (accessed on 30 August 2006).

Lankshear A, Sheldon T, Maynard A, Smith K (2005). 'Nursing challenges: are changes in the nursing role and skill mix improving patient care?' *Health Policy Matters*, vol 10, July. Available online at: www.york.ac.uk/healthsciences/pubs/Hpm10.pdf (accessed on 30 August 2006).

Maynard A (ed) (2005). *The Public-Private Mix for Health: plus ca change, plus ca meme chose?* Oxford and Seattle: Radcliffe Publishing and the Nuffield Trust.

Maynard A, Bloor K (2003). 'Do those who pay the piper call the tune?' *Health Policy Matters*, vol 8, October. Available online at: www.york.ac.uk/healthsciences/pubs/hpm8final.pdf (accessed on 30 August 2006).

Maynard A, Sheldon T (2002). 'Funding the National Health Service'. *Lancet*, vol 360, p 576.

Office of Fair Trading (2006). 'OFT to continue study into drug pricing scheme'. Press Release 59/06, 23 March, London. Available online at: www.oft.gov.uk?News/Press+releases/2006/59-06.htm (accessed on 30 August 2006).

Reinhardt U (1982). 'Table manners at the health care feast' in *Financing Health Care: Competition versus regulation*, Yaggy D and Anylan WA eds. Cambridge, MA: Ballinger.

Stevens S (2004). 'Reform strategies for the English NHS'. *Health Affairs*, vol 23, 3, pp 37–44.

Stoddart G, Barer M, Evans RG (1994). *User Charges, Snares and Delusions: Another look at the literature*. Ontario: Premier's Council on Health, Well-being and Justice.

Timmins N (2006). 'NHS faces spending squeeze', *Financial Times*, 17 January.

Williams A (1998). 'Medicine, ethics, economics and the National Health Service: a clash of cultures?' In *Radicalism and Reality in the NHS: Fifty years and more*, Bloor K ed. York: University of York.

Yates J (1995). *Private Eye, Heart and Hip*. London: Churchill Livingstone.

Health and the public spending squeeze
Funding prospects for the NHS

Robert Chote

Health and the public spending squeeze
Funding prospects for the NHS

Robert Chote

Introduction

Over the past seven years, the National Health Service (NHS) has enjoyed its largest sustained increase in spending since its inception in 1949. Average real increases of 7.1 per cent a year have lifted health spending from 5.4 per cent of national income in 1998/9 to an estimated 7.2 per cent of national income in 2005/6. Health has been the biggest beneficiary of Gordon Brown's years of plenty, accounting for nearly 40 per cent of the total increase in public spending as a share of national income over this period.

But the pace of growth in overall public spending is already slowing, and the Chancellor of the Exchequer has pencilled in figures showing a further deceleration over the period to be covered by the 2007 Comprehensive Spending Review (CSR) – from 2008/9 to 2010/1. But will the Chancellor be as tough as his Budget figures suggest? And, if he is, how much of the pain might the NHS be expected to bear?

The public finances and the looming spending squeeze

The Chancellor's decisions on tax and spending are (in principle) constrained by his fiscal rules: the *golden rule* requires him to borrow only to invest on average over the ups and downs of the economic cycle (and thus to keep the current Budget in balance or surplus); the *sustainable investment rule* requires him to keep public sector net debt below 40 per cent of national income in every year of the current economic cycle.

Four or five years ago, it looked as though the rules would be met with a huge margin to spare over the cycle that the Treasury then expected to span the seven financial years from 1999/2000 to 2005/6 – even though the Chancellor had decided to increase public spending rapidly, following the initial years of restraint when he stuck to the plans he inherited from the Conservatives. But while spending duly rose significantly as a share of national income during Labour's second term, tax revenues weakened suddenly and unexpectedly in 2001/2 and 2002/3 as a falling stock market hit City profits and bonuses – a fruitful source of revenue for the Treasury.

In successive Budgets and Pre-Budget Reports, the Chancellor predicted that corporation tax payments in particular were about to rebound. But his forecasts were consistently overoptimistic. Ahead of the 2005 general election, the Institute for Fiscal Studies and other analysts argued that the Treasury's forecasts for revenues and government borrowing were about 1 per cent of national income (£121/2 billion in today's money) too optimistic at the end of its five-year forecasting horizon. We argued that the Chancellor should adopt more cautious revenue forecasts and that some combination of fresh tax increases and reductions in public spending plans would be necessary to bring about the improvement in the public finances that he thought necessary to meet his fiscal rules with an appropriate degree of caution. He maintained that his forecasts were reasonable and no policy changes were necessary to adhere to the rules.

Shortly after the election, it was clear that government borrowing was once again failing to shrink as quickly as the Treasury had hoped. Indeed, the cumulative effect of five years of forecast downgrades had been to exhaust the Chancellor's room for manoeuvre in meeting the golden rule. In June 2005 the Treasury published figures showing that the current Budget deficit – the shortfall between tax revenues and current (non-investment) spending – was only 10 per cent smaller in the first two months of the 2005/6 financial year than in the equivalent period of 2004/5. If this remained the case, the current Budget deficit would come in at around £15 billion for the year as a whole, rather than the £5.7 billion predicted in the 2005 Budget. The Chancellor would breach the golden rule over the current cycle. Such a breach would probably have little direct economic impact, but it would certainly be embarrassing for Mr Brown.

A month later, the Treasury conveniently published a paper noting that economic activity had been slightly stronger than it had previously thought in 1999, and arguing that the current economic cycle had thus begun in 1997/8 rather than 1999/2000. At a stroke this made the golden rule easier to meet, because the government had run a significant current Budget surplus in 1998/9. Pushing back the start of the cycle increased the amount the Chancellor could borrow for the current Budget in 2005/6 without breaking the golden rule from £9.6 billion to £22.5 billion.

The case for beginning the cycle in 1997/8 was not unreasonable, but it was less powerful that it would have been at any time over the previous three years. By making the change at precisely the point at which it was necessary to get the government back on course to meet the golden rule, the Chancellor undermined the credibility of his fiscal pledges. It could now be suggested – rightly or wrongly – that he was ready to move the goalposts if and when it was necessary to avoid an embarrassing breach of the rules.

In the Pre-Budget Report of December 2005, the Chancellor further announced that he expected the current economic cycle to end in 2008/9 rather than 2005/6. The Treasury predicted that the government would run a very small current Budget surplus on average over these three years, so this again boosted the margin with which he expected the golden rule to be met. However, this change in date also increases the uncertainty around the forecasts. In line with the advice that we and others gave him before the election, he also reduced his underlying corporation tax revenue forecasts, announced £3 billion of tax increases (mostly on North Sea oil companies) and pencilled in a cut in public spending as a share of national income for the period to be covered by the 2007 CSR. For the third parliamentary term running, the Chancellor chose to make a painful fiscal adjustment in the 12 months following an election.

By the standards of the Pre-Budget Report, the 2006 Budget was – on first inspection – a non-event. The Chancellor made few changes to his forecasts for the economy and public

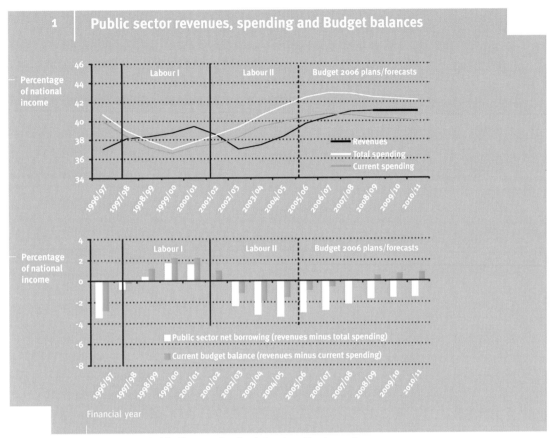

1 Public sector revenues, spending and Budget balances

Source: HM Treasury, *Public Finances Databank*, London, March 2006,
www.hm-treasury.gov.uk/media/415/DC/psfmarch2006.xls (accessed on 30 August 2006)

finances, and announced no significant net giveaway or fiscal tightening. He continued to pencil in a tightening squeeze on public spending from 2008/9 and signalled his intent by pre-announcing tough settlements for five Whitehall departments. So what do the Budget projections imply for the outlook for the public finances and spending?

As Figure 1 above illustrates, the Treasury expects the current Budget balance to move from a deficit of 0.9 per cent of national income last year to a surplus of 0.8 per cent of national income in 2010/1. This would meet the golden rule with £10.1 billion to spare, over the newly elongated 12-year cycle ending in 2008/9. (The Chancellor quoted £16 billion in his Budget speech by assuming that his 'rainy day' reserve will remain unspent.)

On the revenue side, there are two main risks to this scenario. First, there may be less spare capacity in the economy than the Treasury thinks, and therefore less scope for the economy (and tax revenues) to grow before the cycle comes to an end. Second, tax revenues could fail to grow as quickly as the Treasury hopes for any given state of the economy. Either risk could imperil the Chancellor's hopes of meeting the golden rule in this cycle and leave the public finances weaker than expected going into the next. We remain a little more pessimistic than the Treasury about the path of revenues over the next five years, but to a much smaller degree than a year ago. Given the uncertainty that inevitably surrounds the outlook for the public finances over even a short time horizon, there seems little reason to alter significantly our judgement in January that the Chancellor has a roughly 50/50 chance of meeting the rule on current policies.

Another risk cited by some commentators is that the economy may simply perform more weakly than expected in the short term. However, if that creates more spare capacity, the economy could grow more strongly in the longer term to make up the lost ground. This would certainly be awkward for Mr Brown, by depressing tax revenues and pushing up borrowing in the short term. Nevertheless, the Chancellor could reasonably expect to recover the lost revenues later when the economy recovers. Both the letter and the spirit of his fiscal rules allow the government to borrow more when the economy is temporarily weak, as long as offsetting surpluses are accumulated when the economy is unsustainably strong. Allowing 'automatic stabilisers' to work in this way can help stabilise the economy.

Even if these risks do not materialise, the improvement in the public finances that the Chancellor projects over the next five years depends on his 'inking in' the spending figures that he has so far pencilled in for the period covered by the CSR.

As Figure 2 opposite illustrates, the Treasury projections assume that the slowdown in spending growth already underway in Spending Review 2004 (covering 2005/6 to 2007/8) intensifies thereafter. Public spending is assumed to rise by only 1.9 per cent a year on average in real terms in the three years 2008/9 to 2010/1. This is less than half the 4.1 per cent a year increase expected in the preceding nine years from 1999/2000. Spending growth will only have been weaker in Labour's first three years in office, when the party was sticking to the plans it inherited from the Conservatives, or when departments were underspending their budgets in 1999/2000. The projected growth rate of 1.9 per cent a year is also slower than the growth rate of the economy, reducing spending from 43.1 per cent of national income in 2007/8 to 42.5 per cent of national income in 2010/1. But this would still reverse only a small part of the rise since 1999/2000.

The Chancellor has warned that the projections used in the Budget are not necessarily those that he will adopt as firm plans, which he is expected to announce in Budget 2007. But how plausible are these numbers? Broadly speaking, he has three options: stick to the projections; spend more and tax more; or spend more and borrow more.

Stick to the projections The CSR 2007 period will almost certainly span the date of the next general election, which must take place by the early summer of 2010. It is obviously not ideal for the Chancellor – who presumably hopes to be Prime Minister by then – to fight a general election in the midst of a public spending squeeze. But tough public spending plans would also limit the Conservatives' room for manoeuvre. If Mr Brown is already squeezing spending, it is less plausible for the Conservatives to propose an even tighter squeeze to finance tax cuts without raising additional fears for the quality of public services. It is perhaps more likely that the Conservatives would promise to stick to the government's spending plans in their initial years in office, as Labour did in 1997.

Spend more and tax more The Chancellor and his entourage are proud of the fact that they secured public acceptance for a significant tax increase (around £8 billion) in the 2002 Budget by arguing that this would pay for greater investment in the NHS (although it could just as plausibly have been described as additional money for tax credits). Mr Brown could attempt the same again. He would need to raise a similar amount

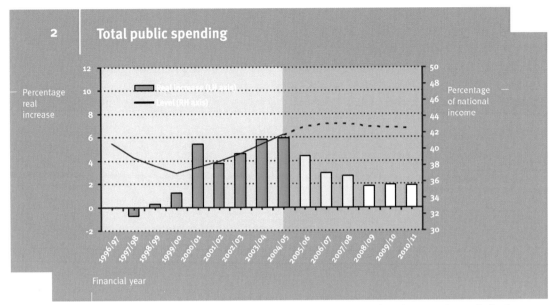

Percentage real increase

Percentage of national income

Real increase (LH axis)
Level (RH axis)

Financial year

Note: Growth in real spending is calculated by deflating spending by growth in the Gross Domestic Product (GDP) deflator. Although this might not be the appropriate deflator for the increase in the cost of goods and services purchased by public spending, it could be considered the most appropriate deflator when looking at the cost to the taxpayer.

Source: HM Treasury, *Budget 2006*,
www.hm-treasury.gov.uk/budget/budget_06/budget_report/bud_bud06_repindex.cfm
(accessed on 30 August 2006)

as in 2002 (0.7 per cent of national income) to stabilise public spending as a share of national income across CSR 2007 rather than reduce it. However, the tax burden has already risen by 2.1 per cent of national income since 2002/3 and the Treasury expects it to rise by a further 1.2 per cent of national income by 2010/1 on 'existing policies'. Selling a further tax increase might therefore be rather more difficult than in 2002.

Spend more and borrow more The Chancellor could choose to spend more and finance it by higher borrowing rather than by tax increases. But extra borrowing in 2008/9 would make the golden rule more difficult to meet in the current economic cycle, while extra borrowing in 2009/10 and 2010/1 would make it more difficult to meet in the next (assuming that the dating of the cycle does not change again). There is the additional problem that the sustainable investment rule is now becoming increasingly binding. The Budget forecast a public sector net debt of 38.4 per cent of national income in 2010/1, just 1.6 per cent of national income below the ceiling. Borrowing more to keep public spending growing in line with the economy over the three years of CSR 2007 would eliminate this cushion almost entirely. Of course, the Chancellor could choose to 'move the goalposts' in some way to make life easier for himself, but given the loss of credibility he appears to have suffered following the recent re-dating of the cycle, this might appear unduly risky.

Once the Chancellor has announced the overall spending envelope, he will have to decide how it is to be shared across departments, although in practice the overall spending totals and the outcome for key spending areas will be decided in tandem. We now discuss how health might fare relative to other spending priorities if the Chancellor sticks with his provisional spending totals.

Health spending: a winner or a loser?

The Chancellor's Budget speech gave some interesting clues to the likely shape of the CSR. Concretely, Mr Brown announced that Home Office spending would be frozen in real terms and that spending by the Department for Work and Pensions (not including the bulk of social security spending), HM Treasury, HM Revenue & Customs and the Cabinet Office would be cut by 5 per cent a year in real terms.

These are relatively small beer, together accounting for less than 6 per cent of total public spending. If spending overall rises by 1.9 per cent a year in real terms, these settlements imply that the remainder can rise by 2.1 per cent a year in real terms – still lower than the growth rate of the economy and smaller than the increases seen in recent years.

In addition to these concrete numbers, the Chancellor sent a potentially interesting signal in his Budget speech by talking at length about the need to increase spending per pupil in education and not at all about the NHS – which has of course been plagued with politically embarrassing financial difficulties. Does this suggest that, while the NHS fared even better than education during the years of plenty, Mr Brown might see education as the higher priority during the years of stringency?

If so, how might these two traditional Labour priorities trade off against each other? To judge this, we need to make illustrative assumptions about spending elsewhere.

Overseas development assistance We can be fairly confident that overseas aid will do well in the spending review. The 2005 Labour Party manifesto promised to increase it to the United Nations (UN) target of 0.7 per cent of national income by 2013. If the government makes steady progress towards this objective, it will need to increase aid spending by 10.4 per cent a year in real terms.

Social security benefits and tax credits Since Labour came to power, spending on social security benefits and tax credits has grown on average by 2.2 per cent a year in real terms. The government does not lay down three-year plans for these areas, leaving them to be 'annually managed' within the overall envelope. But it seems reasonable to assume that the spending in these areas will grow at least as strongly looking forward – the government is already falling behind its targets for child poverty, unemployment is rising and the Chancellor also hinted that the forthcoming pensions White Paper would give more to current pensioners. Conversely, the Treasury doubtless hopes to make savings by making reforms to incapacity benefits.

Other non-education and non-health spending To give the government scope to be as generous as possible to health and education, we assume that other spending is frozen in real terms. This could be tough to achieve, as it includes the politically sensitive transport budget. It also includes defence, which has been a source of savings in recent decades but where pressures in Iraq and Afghanistan have forced the government to find extra money.

Having made these assumptions, let us further assume that Mr Brown wishes to increase health spending by the minimum 4.4 per cent a year in real terms recommended by the

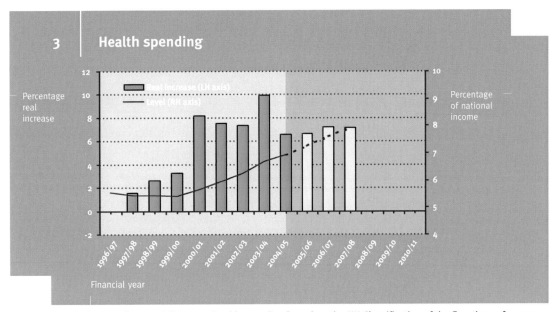

3 | Health spending

Notes: Figures refer to public sector health spending based on the UN Classification of the Functions of Government (COFOG), the international standard, as used in the Public Expenditure Statistical Analysis. Growth in real health spending is calculated by deflating spending by growth in the GDP deflator. Although this might not be the appropriate deflator for the increase in the cost of goods and services purchased by health spending, it could be considered the most appropriate deflator when looking at the cost to the taxpayer.

Sources: Period to 2004/5 from HM Treasury, *Latest Functional Data*, July 2005, www.hm-treasury.gov.uk/media/344/99/latest_functional_tables_peowp05.xls; period from 2005/6 onwards from table 8.2 of HM Treasury, *2004 Spending Review: Stability, Security and Opportunity for All: Investing for Britain's Long-Term Future: New Public Spending Plans 2005–2008*, Cm. 6327, 2004, www.hm-treasury.gov.uk/spending_review/spend_sr04/report/spend_sr04_repindex.cfm

Wanless Report (the 'fully engaged' scenario). As Figure 3 above illustrates, this would be well below the 7.1 per cent a year it has been allocated in previous spending reviews. The Chancellor would then be able to increase education spending by only 3.4 per cent a year, well below the 5.6 per cent a year it has been allocated in previous spending reviews.

Mr Brown has said, however, that he is re-examining the need for extra spending identified by the Wanless Report – presumably not in the expectation that he will come up with an even higher figure (although the International Monetary Fund and others have argued that the Treasury is underestimating the long-term upward pressure on health spending from technological advances and demands as people's incomes rise). If the Chancellor wished to maintain the past pace of growth in education spending at 5.6 per cent a year, health spending could rise by only 2.8 per cent a year. But he might well be unwilling to reduce growth in health spending below the 3.1 per cent a year it averaged under the Conservatives between 1979 and 1997, in which case education spending could grow by 5.2 per cent a year.

Needless to say, if the Chancellor wished to be more generous in areas such as transport and defence, the available resources for health and education would be reduced. Conversely, if he decides to increase the overall spending envelope from the figures published in the Budget, he could be more generous.

1 | **Illustrative trade-offs between health and education in percentage increase in spending**

	I	II	III
Health	2.8%	3.1% (Tories 1979–97)	4.4% (Wanless minimum)
Education	5.6% (Labour Spending Reviews to date)	5.2%	3.4%

Note: Assumes real spending growth of 0% per annum for the Home Office, −5% for Department for Work & Pensions, HM Treasury, HM Revenue & Customs and the Cabinet Office, 10.4% for overseas development assistance, 2.2% for social security and tax credits, and 0% for other spending.

Conclusion

Public spending has moved through three distinct phases under Gordon Brown's Chancellorship: a tight squeeze as he built fiscal credibility by sticking to the plans he inherited from the Conservatives; rapid increases as he pumped money into health, education and tax credits; and now gradual retrenchment as he tries to reduce government borrowing after a succession of overoptimistic fiscal forecasts.

Health was the big winner during the years of plenty, with education not far behind. Both would expect to see some reduction in generosity now that the overall spending envelope is tightening. But Mr Brown's Budget speech has raised the additional possibility that he will see education, rather than health, as the top priority.

When is enough, and how do we know?

Spending on health care

John Appleby

When is enough, and how do we know?
Spending on health care

John Appleby[1]

Introduction

In 2000, Prime Minister Tony Blair committed his government to increasing health spending as a proportion of Gross Domestic Product (GDP) up to the average level in the European Union (Appleby and Boyle 2000). In line with that commitment, the National Health Service (NHS) budget has been growing at around 10 per cent a year – around 7.5 per cent in real (GDP-deflated) terms. These are unprecedented growth rates. If maintained, it would mean that by 2008 total (public plus private[2]) spending on health care would absorb around 9.8 per cent of GDP – equivalent to spending levels in France in 2001.

If spending increased at the same rate beyond 2008, by 2011 spending would have risen to around 11 per cent of GDP – similar to German levels in 2001. In a further five or six years, total UK health care spending would reach levels similar to those currently committed by the highest-spending country in the world: the United States (*see* Figure 1 overleaf).

Growth already committed represents a massive increase – equivalent to around 2.5 percentage points of GDP between 1997 and 2007. This commitment reflects a political judgement about the kind and quality of health care England should enjoy. It had been apparent for some time that the performance of the NHS in comparison with other European health care systems was poor, particularly with respect to access – waiting times for operations and for seeing hospital specialists were perhaps the longest in Europe – but also with respect to clinical outcomes. Comparative studies of cancer survival rates also showed England to be below the European average on some key cancers (Coleman *et al* 2003). The need to spend more, particularly to increase the numbers of clinical staff, seemed inescapable.

The scale of the required increase had been estimated in reports commissioned by the Chancellor from Derek Wanless and his team within the Treasury. These assessed the likely costs of a future NHS in which waiting times had been virtually eradicated, productivity increased, quality programmes developed and maintained across all health care activities, and the population fully engaged with public health messages and judicious use of health care to maximise their own health (Wanless 2002).

---

1 This presentation is based on Appleby J, Harrison A (2006). Spending on Health: How much is enough? London: King's Fund.
2 Assuming private spending to remain constant at around 1.2 per cent of GDP.

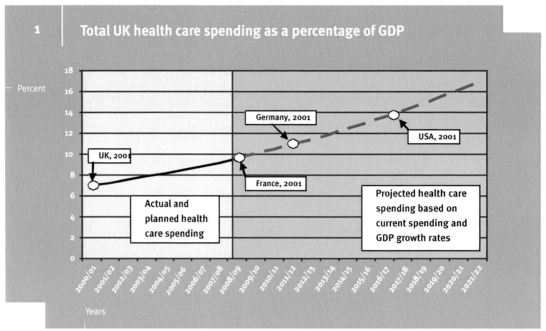

1 | **Total UK health care spending as a percentage of GDP**

Percent

Germany, 2001

USA, 2001

UK, 2001

France, 2001

Actual and
planned health
care spending

Projected health care
spending based on
current spending and
GDP growth rates

Years

Source: Authors' calculations

Although this pragmatic approach to defining spending levels had the merit of defining the need for a major increase in spending, it suffered from three significant weaknesses.

■ First, it did not explicitly or systematically[3] demonstrate what health benefits the additional resources proposed by the Wanless Report would produce, nor whether those resources could produce more health benefits in other non-health care uses (such as education or poverty reduction – both of which are known to be linked to health).

■ Second, it did not consider in detail whether there were other means of producing the improved health outcomes that the extra spending produced. One of the options developed, termed the 'fully engaged' scenario, did suggest that a rebalancing towards public health measures would be more effective in cost and health outcome terms, but this was not investigated in depth at the time. A subsequent report (Wanless 2004) reaffirmed the potential of public health measures, but lack of evidence ruled out development of the scenario into a plan of action.

■ Third, it did not consider what would follow *after* the target performance levels had been achieved. Implicitly, meeting them would mean that the NHS was 'good enough': but by the time that they were forecast to be achieved, the forces making for increased spending – principally improvements in medical technology – would almost certainly have created new spending opportunities.

The recommendations of the first Wanless Report remain in force: the existing spending plans will carry through to 2007/8. But what after that? Wanless suggested that, in two of his three future scenarios, spending should plateau at around 10.5 to just over 11 per cent

---

3 Although some estimates of benefits (in terms of lives saved) of some components of the extra spending were suggested explicitly (eg, for increased spending to improve clinical governance) and implicitly as a result of implementing National Service Frameworks for coronary heart disease, no estimates were made in areas such as extra spending required to reduce waiting times (a significant proportion of the total extra spend recommended), and no attempt was made to present benefits in a commensurate form (such as quality-adjusted life years).

of GDP by 2022, and for the third, should tend to a limit of just over 14 per cent after this date. But he offered little justification for proposing these turning points. Indeed, the only justification given was that by around 2022 UK health care spending will have 'caught up' with its European neighbours and that spending decisions after this merely become a question of 'keeping up' (*see* Figure 2 below).

However, if health spending continued to grow at current rates, by 2026 the UK could be spending one pound in every five in the economy on health care. Stretching such projections to their limit, in 40 years' time, half the nation's wealth would be spent on health care. To accommodate such spending, consumption of non-health care goods and services as a proportion of GDP would have to decline massively (although, assuming continuation of historic trends in the expansion of the economy as a whole, real expenditure in this sector would actually increase). Taxes would in all likelihood have to rise (with increases ameliorated somewhat because of the larger tax pool) and other public services would see their share of GDP decline (although, again, real spending could still increase). Furthermore, health employment would rise substantially and productivity in the economy overall would fall as the traditionally lower levels of productivity growth of the health sector dilute higher levels in other sectors of the economy. Such projections have been made for the US health care system (Technical Review Panel 2000) and been regarded as sustainable, even desirable (Fogel 2004).

To a British government – and particularly a Labour one – such projections are the stuff of nightmares. For over half a century the UK has operated a two-tier health care system: the rich have always been able to buy care from the private sector and thus bypass the long queues within the NHS. This explains why, despite a raft of initiatives targeted at improving clinical quality, reducing access times has been the dominant health policy

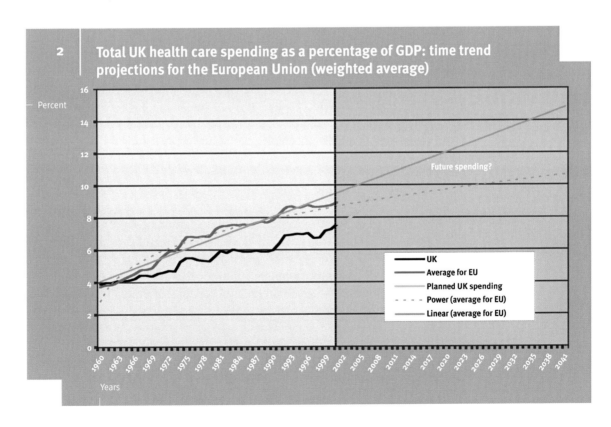

2 | **Total UK health care spending as a percentage of GDP: time trend projections for the European Union (weighted average)**

goal since Labour came to power (Harrison and Appleby 2005). The present government is aiming for a one-tier system in which the NHS increases its market (monopoly) position in part by matching private sector performance (particularly on waiting times) and in part by expanding its (increasingly monopsonistic) purchasing of privately provided care on behalf of NHS patients.

But pursuit of this goal has proved expensive – and despite significant achievements, it is still not achieved. As a result the government will soon face a very awkward dilemma: if it continues to aim for an NHS free to all and that all want to use, this would seem to require yet more years of rapid expenditure growth. But other claims on the public purse are also growing, particularly education, pensions and social care for the elderly. And while the fiscal position for the past ten years has been strong, the government is now faced with a relative decline in economic performance and a deteriorating fiscal position.

Although the Treasury foot is poised over the health care spending brake, it seems very likely that the pressures to spend more will continue to grow more rapidly than the projected budget could cope with. If this is the case, the question will arise as to whether the forces making for more spending should be resisted or whether they should be accommodated by making more finance available, either through existing means such as general taxation, or in some other way.

In this paper we focus on the analytical framework in which answers to these questions can best be addressed. First, we examine why health care spending tends to grow; then the reasons for limiting health care spending; and finally, accepting that limits are inevitable, how these might be arrived at in a publicly funded health care system.

Why does health care spending grow?

The case for resisting further rapid expenditure growth rests in part on the factors lying behind it. If, for example, changes in demography were largely responsible, then it would be hard to argue that it should be resisted – if it was, then average standards of care would fall unless offsetting gains in efficiency could be achieved. If, on the other hand, growth was largely accounted for by improvements in the quality and effectiveness of the care available, then the question would be: what rate of improvement is it worthwhile financing (given other calls on scarce public/societal resources)?

Reinhardt et al (2004) have noted in relation to historic US health care growth that ability to pay (as measured by, for example, GDP per capita) explains around 90 per cent of cross-sectional international variation in health care spend, as well as being associated with trends in spending for individual countries – including England. However, this does not explain why health care should be the spending area of choice as national income rises. Furthermore, in the context of determining the NHS budget, although there is a clear and persistent cross-sectional link between GDP and health care spend per capita, there is no a priori reason why the relationship between wealth and health should be used as a normative guide.

The low importance attached to demography runs counter to what has often been assumed in the past. The average age of the population in most countries has been rising and, at an individual level, health spending rises with age, particularly towards the very end of life. But an increase in the general level of health has meant that most of the 'costs of dying' have been postponed and the number of years of healthy life extended. Several studies have suggested that as the average age at death has risen, the associated costs have been postponed.

Using data for England, Seshamani and Gray (2004) found, for example, that proximity to death explained most of the increase in health spending at the end of life. The rest was due to age. Dixon *et al* (2004) found that the average number of bed days spent in hospital in the period before death does not increase with increasing age. Other work (Canadian Health Services Research Foundation 2003) suggests that the older people are when they die, the lower their health care costs tend to be (although their social care costs may be higher). This work suggests that earlier estimates of the health care costs of an ageing population considerably exaggerated the impact of demographic change.[4]

Technological change – new medicines, new surgical techniques etc – is identified as the dominant factor (*see* Figure 3 below); Newhouse (1992) estimates that it accounted for over 65 per cent of the growth in US health spend from 1940 to 1990, while Cutler (1995) provides a lower, but still dominant estimate of 49 per cent. On the other hand, increases in costs are also significant in reducing the value of the gains from new technology. Both studies suggest, however, that income growth has been significant; this suggests that, as people become richer, they are willing to pay more for a given improvement in health – in other words, higher costs (or smaller marginal gains in benefits) may be offset by increases in perceived value.

The accuracy of these estimates is hard to judge; but even harder to judge is the impact future technological development will have on health care spending. New medical technologies can open up brand-new areas for medical intervention and new levels of

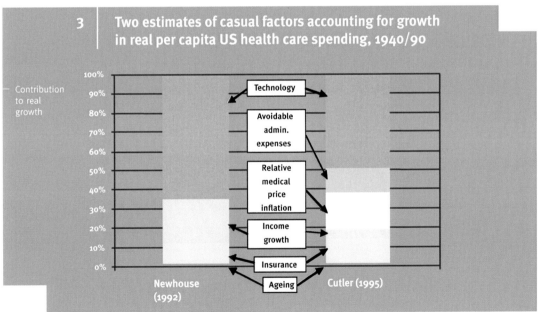

3 | Two estimates of casual factors accounting for growth in real per capita US health care spending, 1940/90

Source: Newhouse (1992) and Cutler (1995)

---

4 It was common practice to estimate the impact of ageing by using per capita spending on each age group in a recent year and applying the resultant figures to estimates of the age structure of the population at some future date.

intensity for existing health care interventions. New medical technologies can be cost-reducing or cost-increasing, but (at least historically, as Newhouse and Cutler suggest) the net impact of technological development on the costs of health care have been not only positive, but the major driver for increased health care spending.

So, should the NHS budget be allowed to expand to keep up with such technical advances? If not, what justification can be provided for constraining Exchequer funding?

Why limit spending?

For most goods and services, these questions would not arise. No one would argue for limiting spending on any other consumption good – from TVs to cabbages. This argument is clearly right for all those forms of health care spending (such as over-the-counter drugs) that people meet themselves. If individuals want more analgesics because they are less tolerant of pain than they used to be, *and they bear the costs of such demand themselves*, then their spending decision is theirs alone. The decision they take will be one in which they will (at least in theory and however imperfectly) balance the benefits and costs of their purchase, subject to the alternative benefits they would have to forgo in order to enjoy the benefits of the analgesics. This, in essence, is an unavoidable (and unexceptional) rationing decision performed in private markets.

Those who pay for health care (taxpayers) are not, at any particular time, the same as those who use the services financed in this way. In any system where the link between contributions and consumption is poor,[5] and in particular taxpayer-funded systems such as the United Kingdom NHS, the state must in effect act as a 'guardian' for taxpayers, ensuring that the funds diverted from personal use to health care are well used. If taxpayers could specifically vote on how much should be spent on health care, a limit could be set in that way.

But what kind of arguments would be relevant to inform such a vote? Voters might wish to set limits for a variety of reasons. For example, some kinds of spending might be judged unethical – some advances in reproductive technology such as human cloning perhaps fall into this category. Equally, some of the purposes of health spending may be questioned. For example, Hanson and Callahan (1999) consider that the case for using medical knowledge to enhance 'natural' human characteristics might be considered an ethical step too far.

Other limits might be desirable because certain services – such as cosmetic surgery (increasingly including dentistry) – may be considered inappropriate for public subsidy and hence not classified as health care, for example. But there are no clear-cut criteria for determining what is or what is not health care. Complementary medicines, 'healthy' foods and activities such as systematic exercise are emerging as potential candidates for extending the scope of publicly funded health care rather than diminishing it.

But perhaps the most important reason for limiting the scope for funding health care is that the benefits of additional spending may be judged insufficient to justify the transfer

---

5 By design in the UK NHS, and often by default in insurance-based systems.

of funds from personal to public use. Although more spending on health arising from the introduction of new medical technologies may provide some benefits, they may be outweighed by the benefits in other uses (that is, the *opportunity costs* of providing them). In principle, therefore, a benefit–cost test applied to all health spending would provide a means of defining when the budget was large enough.[6]

An economic rationalist approach

The NHS has for some time applied a cost-effectiveness approach to resource allocation decisions *within* its overall budget – for example, banning prescribing of therapies deemed clinically ineffective (such as cough remedies). Subsequently, this approach was put on a more systematic footing with the establishment of the National Institute for Health and Clinical Excellence (NICE) in 2005.[7] NICE collects and reviews the evidence bearing on the value of new drugs and other forms of treatment, and issues advice to the NHS as to whether particular interventions should be used. So far it has made very few recommendations to exclude the interventions it has considered, but it has recommended the use of cheaper forms of treatment where more expensive ones are judged to provide little or no extra benefit. In net terms, to date, NICE's guidance has been cost-increasing for the NHS. It should be noted, however, that its recommendations have so far affected only a very small percentage of the total NHS spend per annum.

Although, by consensus, NICE performs an essential function, its main task – the systematic weighing-up of costs and benefits – is one that we argue should be carried out at other levels in the NHS – in particular, as part of an approach to setting limits on health care spending.

The viewpoint we take is thus essentially an economic one: that is, spending on health care, as on any other good, is worthwhile as long as the benefits it brings exceed those that could be obtained by other forms of spending. In other words, it is worth spending more on health as long as the benefits achieved outweigh the *opportunity costs*. Implicit in the recent increases in NHS spending noted earlier is the judgement that, despite the increases that have already occurred in health spending, the benefits continue to be greater in health care than in other possible uses.

The usual assumption, however, is that as spending in a particular area rises, there will inevitably come a point where the benefits at the margin will tend to fall. There may very possibly also be a point after which the absolute benefits fall as spending increases still further.

There is no reason why health should be an exception. At low levels of spending, the most productive activities (in terms of generating health), such as immunisation and vaccination, along with basic primary care and the most cost-effective drugs, will be worth financing. As spending rises, it will tend to be devoted to activities and treatments that, while beneficial, yield less in terms of direct health benefits as conventionally

---

6 The need to focus on the outcomes, and in particular the relationship between the (financial) inputs and (health) outcomes, has been made by others. *See*, for example, Propper (2001).

7 The new Institute combined the National Institute for Clinical Excellence (NICE) and the Health Development Agency (retaining the acronym of the former), expanding its role to cover public health interventions. NICE has been carrying out its work on clinical and cost-effective guidelines since its formation in 1999.

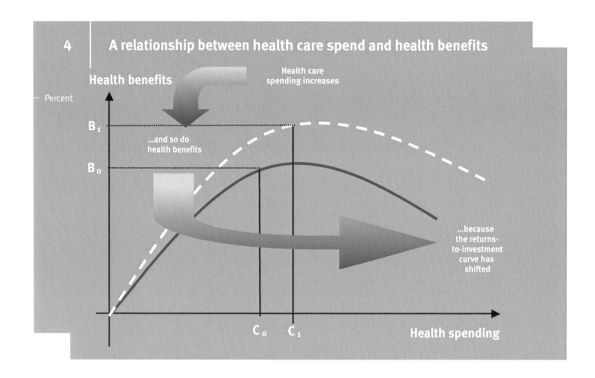

4 **A relationship between health care spend and health benefits**

Health benefits

Percent

Health care spending increases

B₁ ....

...and so do
health benefits

B₀ ....

...because
the returns-
to-investment
curve has
shifted

C₀   C₁

Health spending

measured by, for example, reductions in mortality or increases in life expectancy. Of course, such activities may produce more in other terms, such as convenience of access, a more pleasant care process and so on. Figure 4 above captures this view of diminishing marginal (and total) returns.

The relationship between health care spend and health benefits is not static, and will change over time for four main reasons:

■ the cost of provision may rise or fall so that at every level of spend, more (or less) benefits are produced

■ the nature and extent of ill health in the population may rise, increasing the need for treatment and the potential benefit from spending more

■ the *value* attached to health benefits may rise or fall for a variety of reasons

■ new treatments may be introduced because of technological change; while some may reduce the cost of treatment, others may extend its scope.

While unit cost increases (decreases) shift the curve downwards (upwards), the effect of the second type of change is to extend the curve upwards (for any given level of spend, more benefit is obtained). The effect of the final two changes is indeterminate. The question we now consider is: given current levels of spending and the relationship between spending and health benefits (the shape of the returns-to-investment curve), where on the curve is the UK at the moment?

The flat of the curve?

Given the government's decision to devote extra resources to the NHS, the answer may seem obvious: where the gradient is steep. And, indeed, as Reinhardt *et al* (2004) have assumed, while the US and Canada are presumed to be nearer the flat of their hypothetical quality-adjusted life years (QALY) supply curve, the UK, they suggest, is on the rising part of the curve. Pinning down empirical evidence on this matter is hard. There are macro (country-level) and micro (intervention/disease-level) studies of the returns to health care investment that suggest (and the much more comprehensive reviews such as that by Nolte and McKee [2004] confirm) that there is evidence that health spending has produced a positive return as measured by a variety of health outcomes – life expectancy, reduced mortality etc – but that as spending rises, the rate of health returns tends to fall.

However, it is also clear that there are statistical limits to, first, disentangling the determinants of observed changes in health; and, second, establishing the marginal product of health care (and how this might be changing over time).

In addition, in inter-country comparisons, the measure of the actual *return* (the benefit) to investment has tended to focus on outcomes such as mortality or life expectancy – mainly because these are routinely measured – and tend to ignore other valid reasons for investment – such as improvements in quality of life or the process of health care. Micro- or individual intervention studies (for example, the technology assessments carried out by NICE and some of the 'inventory' approaches such as those by Bunker [2001]) attempt to incorporate a quality-of-life dimension (such as by using weights to calculate QALYs). However, no study to date has managed a comprehensive and unambiguous assessment of the total returns to health care investment – including all sources of benefit and disbenefit.

In relation to the recent large increases in spending in the English NHS, the traditional complaint – where's the money? – has moved on to: where has the money gone? and by extension, what have we got for the extra spending? Answering this last question is extremely difficult. There are measurable benefits – especially in terms of better access and reduced waiting times – but little or no evidence on outcome gains (Appleby and Harrison 2005). But the beneficiaries of the new investment are not always patients. On some estimates, up to three-quarters of the annual cash increases to the NHS over the past few years have been absorbed by pay and price increases and other cost pressures rather than by volume and quality improvements (King's Fund 2005). Owing to the lack of definitive data in many key areas, it is impossible to come to a firm conclusion as to where the NHS (in England) is located on the returns curve. Recent reviews of the performance of the NHS have emphasised how few conclusions can be drawn on whether or not particular services have improved – see, for example, Leatherman and Sutherland (2003) and Healthcare Commission (2004).

From the limited data that does exist, it is hard to demonstrate that the NHS is on the steepest part of the curve where the health returns from additional spending are high. In no area among those reviewed are there major identifiable health gains that can be attributed to extra health spending alone. This is even true of the diseases such as cancer and coronary heart disease (CHD) on which the government has focused extra resources. Improvements have been recorded in survival and mortality rates, but the contribution of NHS expenditure is difficult to isolate from the other factors at work, such as reductions in smoking or dietary change. However, there is recent, qualified, evidence that although two-thirds of the reduction in CHD mortality in Britain between 1981 and 2000 is due to preventive measures, 81 per cent of that reduction is due to 'primary' prevention (changes in lifestyle risk factors such as smoking) and just 19 per cent due to 'secondary' prevention (that is, targeting patients with known CHD) (Unal *et al* 2005[8]). Nonetheless, the main NHS CHD strategy – and significant funding – has been on the latter, where returns (reductions in mortality) appear to be relatively low.

Gains are being achieved in such areas as convenience and process benefits (for example, the changes that have led to shorter waiting times within hospital accident and emergency departments). Some of these may lead to better health outcomes, but the main argument used by the government for setting targets such as these derives from the perception that 'expectations' of service performance are rising and that people want choice of when and where to be treated and easier access to whatever services they choose. While this is intuitively convincing, in fact there is very little hard evidence about the *value* placed on benefits of these kinds, nor indeed of the costs of providing these benefits.

As we showed above, the government has used comparisons with other European countries as a justification for increased spending. But once the existing spending plans have been fulfilled, the case for more spending will have to be made on the basis of the benefits expected to accrue from it.

Up to now the government has resisted this conclusion. It has continued to set ambitious targets for reducing waiting times and improving access to care more generally, for improving the physical environment in which care is provided, and for raising clinical quality of care for major diseases and patient groups. These are all good things to do, but these programmes have not been costed, so the implications for future spending are unknown, and none has been assessed in terms of the benefits it will generate.

As a former ministerial and prime-ministerial health adviser has described, the government has adopted a series of strategies designed to raise the efficiency with which the NHS uses the resources at its disposal (Stevens 2004). Although these have led to some detectable local improvements, the only available measures of NHS productivity suggest that it has declined since its budget started to expand rapidly. This may reflect the inadequacy of the available measures, but in part it also reflects the uncomfortable facts that NHS employees – particularly primary- and secondary-care doctors – have benefited substantially from the increased budget and that, where services have improved, the change has usually taken the form of quality improvements rather than cost reductions.

The government has also taken a number of initiatives designed to reduce the burden of ill-health, including screening programmes, case management of the chronically ill, and dietary and other lifestyle advice, aimed particularly at the young and disadvantaged groups. But these have yet to show any substantial impact and they are in any case working against the tide of rising obesity, higher rates of drug and alcohol use and other risk factors.

---

8 The evidence from this study could be interpreted to suggest not that the NHS was near the flat of the (CHD) curve, but that there was a failure in technical efficiency (although there is a question of the degree of influence that organised health care has over such lifestyle risk factors as smoking).

What should be done?

From Her Majesty's Treasury's viewpoint, it would be desirable to limit the growth of public spending on health care to something near to the rate of growth in the economy as a whole: a level that would be fiscally sustainable. Given the unpredictable nature of technical progress in medicine, that could only be a guideline rather than a hard and fast rule. If major advances in medical technology produced substantial benefits, then the publicly funded system would have to respond.

In the absence of satisfactory measures of the benefits of additional spending, however, any guideline will be impossible to defend. It is therefore essential that the Department of Health carries out or commissions the technical work required to base judgements on the value of new spending programmes.

That will not be effective on its own. Within the current policy framework, key actors in the health care system (and those with an interest in its spending power) operate within a system of incentives which, from the point of view of health care spending, tend to add to pressures to increase spending. To the patients themselves, NHS services are largely free,[9] while those working within the NHS tend to press for more funding when shortfalls in performance are identified or where opportunities for improving services such as the provision of new drugs are identified. Outside the NHS, the pharmaceutical industry is well versed in the skills required to encourage sales of its products, and the media are quick to pick up on any failings on the part of the NHS and attribute them to shortage of funding.

To counter such pressures, however, would require a major reorientation in the way that health policy is developed. Currently the government itself actively encourages easier access to services, without apparently considering the extra demand that this is likely to generate. The government is introducing new policies such as patient choice of hospital without acknowledging that they might carry an opportunity cost that may not be worth the value of the benefits they generate. The combined effect of these and other initiatives is to fuel patient expectations without regard to the cost of meeting them.

England is not the only country to feel the need to set limits to spending. In most countries, the debate has centred on what should or should not be within the publicly funded health care package. But as we have tried to show, the issues run deeper than that. Any attempt to define a sustainable, publicly funded health care system runs counter to *'the notion that all progress is affordable, that all progress brings benefit and increased equality of outcome, and that there is a moral duty to pursue progress'* (Callahan 1999, p 252). These are the deep-seated notions that must be challenged before an effective debate can begin.

---

9 Most English patients have to pay for dental and eye care services, and a charge is levied for prescription drugs. However, exemptions are extensive, and as a result about 85 per cent of prescription drugs attract no charge. Prescription charges in Wales and Scotland are set to be phased out over the next few years.

References

Appleby J, Boyle S (2000). 'Blair's billions: where will he find the money?'. *British Medical Journal*, vol 320, pp 865–67.

Appleby J, Harrison A (2005). *When is Enough Enough, and How do We Know? Setting limits to health spending*. London: King's Fund.

Bunker JP (2001). *Medicine Matters After All: Measuring the benefits of medical care, a healthy lifestyle, and a just social environment*. London: The Nuffield Trust.

Callahan D (1999). *False Hopes: Overcoming the obstacles to a sustainable, affordable medicine*. New Brunswick, NJ: Rutgers University Press.

Canadian Health Services Research Foundation (2003). *Myth: The cost of dying is an increasing strain on the healthcare system*. Ottawa: CHSRF.

Coleman MP, Gatta G, Verdecchia A, Esteve J, Sant M, Storm H, Allemani C, Ciccolallo L, Santaquilani M, Berrino F (2003). 'EUROCARE-3 summary: Cancer survival in Europe at the end of the 20th century'. *Annals of Oncology*, vol 14 (Supplement 5): v128–v149.

Cutler DM (1995). *Technology, health costs, and the NIH*. Harvard University and the National Bureau of Economic Research. Paper prepared for the National Institutes of Health Economics Roundtable on Biomedical Research, Cambridge, MA.

Dixon T, Shaw M, Frankel S, Ebrahim S (2004). 'Hospital admissions, age and death: retrospective cohort study'. *British Medical Journal*, vol 328, pp 1288–90.

Fogel WR (2004). *The Escape from Hunger and Premature Death, 1700–2100: Europe, America and the Third World*. Cambridge Studies in Population, Economy & Society in Past Time. p 95. Cambridge: Cambridge University Press.

Hanson MJ, Callahan D (1999). *The Goals of Medicine*. Washington, DC: Georgetown University Press.

Harrison A, Appleby J (2005).*The War on Waiting for Hospital Treatment: What has Labour achieved and what challenges remain?* London: King's Fund.

Healthcare Commission (2004). *State of Healthcare Report*. London: Healthcare Commission.

King's Fund (2005). *An Independent Audit of the NHS under Labour (1997–2005)*. London: King's Fund.

Leatherman S, Sutherland K (2003). *The Quest for Quality in the NHS: A mid-term evaluation of the ten-year quality agenda*. London: The Stationery Office.

Newhouse JP (1992). 'Medical care costs: how much welfare loss?'. *Journal of Economic Perspectives*, vol 6 (3), pp 3–21.

Nolte E, McKee M (2004). *Does Healthcare Save Lives? Avoidable mortality revisited*. London: The Nuffield Trust.

Propper C (2001). *Expenditure on health care in the UK: A review of the issues*. CMPO Working Paper, University of Bristol.

Reinhardt U, Hussey PS, Anderson GF (2004). 'U.S. health care spending in an international context'. *Health Affairs*, vol 23 (3), 10–25.

Seshamani M, Gray A (2004). 'Ageing and health-care expenditure: the red herring argument revisited'. *Health Economics,* vol 13, pp 303–14.

Stevens S (2004). 'Reform strategies for the English NHS'. *Health Affairs*, vol 23 (3), pp 37–44.

Technical Review Panel on the Medicare Trustees Reports (2000). *Review of Assumptions and Methods of the Medicare Trustees' Financial Projections.* Available online at: www.cms.hhs.gov/ReportsTrustFunds/downloads/TechnicalPanelReport2000.pdf (accessed on 30 August 2006).

Unal B, Critchley JA, Capewell S (2005). 'Modelling the decline in coronary heart disease deaths in England and Wales, 1981–2000: comparing contributions from primary prevention and secondary prevention'. *British Medical Journal*, vol 331, p 614.

Wanless D (2004). *Securing Good Health for the Whole Population. Final Report.* London: HM Treasury.

Wanless D (2002). *Securing Our Future Health: Taking a long-term view. Final Report.* London: HM Treasury.

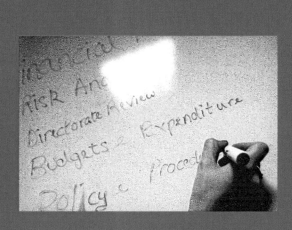

Part 2

Specific issues concerning the Comprehensive Spending Review

Key questions

- What are the future health policy challenges?
- What opportunities are there for demand reduction?
- What scope is there for efficiencies and where can these best be made?
- How can pay best be controlled?

A bigger bang for your buck
Prospects for improving health care productivity

Andy McKeon

A bigger bang for your buck
Prospects for improving health care productivity

Andy McKeon

The current state of NHS productivity

Measurement of National Health Service (NHS) productivity is contentious. At least three different measures have been put forward:

- a 'traditional' measure largely related to the (weighted) number of hospital treatments; on this measure, NHS productivity has fallen by 1.5 per cent a year since 1999

- a quality-adjusted measure from the National Institute for Economic and Social Research (York/NIESR), which would have productivity broadly flat over the same period

- an Office of National Statistics quality-adjusted measure, which would suggest productivity growth of around 1.5 per cent a year.

It is clearly right that productivity measures should address quality as well as quantity. But there are many arguments to be had about whether further quality adjustments can or should be made. The public have, quite literally, paid their money and must now take their choice about how much they have got for it.

The vigour of the debate, however, is explained by the concern that a great deal of money has been invested, particularly in pay deals and additional staff, and that there is not enough progress to show for it. Moreover, there have been clear signals from government that the rate of growth in expenditure on the NHS will slow significantly after 2007/8, reducing from the current annual rate of 7.5 per cent or so in real terms to much less – perhaps 3 per cent or even less. The hunt is on for productivity improvements and greater efficiency in the use of resources so that the service can make the most of the investment it has had, and keep pace with rising demand and expectations. Whatever the arguments about past productivity and its measurement, the simple point is that (a lot) more of it is required in the future.

The scope for achieving greater productivity is well known, through, for example:

- reductions in variation in hospital costs and performance (*see* Figure 1 overleaf)

- reductions in variation of consultant output (*see* Figure 2 overleaf)

- comparison with and convergence towards best practice overseas, with particular examples from Kaiser in the United States where, for example, admission rates can be much lower, particularly for chronic conditions (*see* Table 1, p 65)

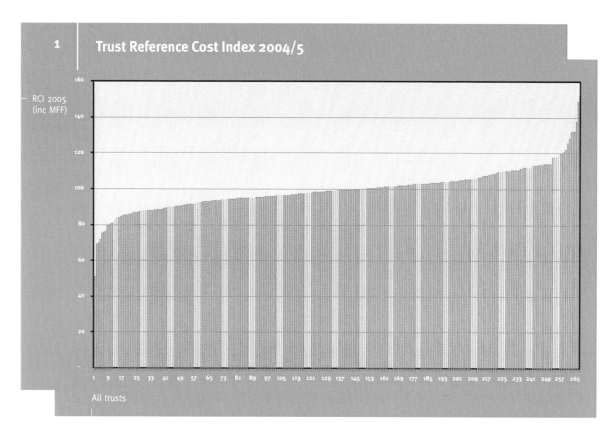

1 | Trust Reference Cost Index 2004/5

RCI 2005
(inc MFF)

All trusts

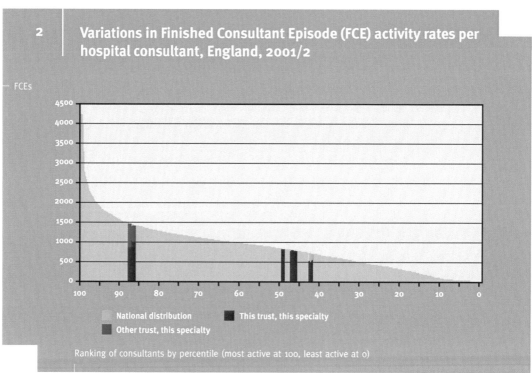

2 | Variations in Finished Consultant Episode (FCE) activity rates per hospital consultant, England, 2001/2

FCEs

National distribution · This trust, this specialty
Other trust, this specialty

Ranking of consultants by percentile (most active at 100, least active at 0)

Source: Ranked activity (FCEs) per consultant in general surgery, 2001/2 data
Anonymous NHS Trust

1 | **Number of inpatient admissions (per 100,000 population) in people aged over 65**

Condition	NHS	Kaiser	
		Unstandardised	Standardised
Stroke	823	712	788
Chronic obstructive pulmonary disease	699	536	558
Bronchitis/asthma	531	129	141
Coronary bypass	144	103	97
Acute myocardial infarction	550	836	893
Heart failure/shock	556	1008	1118
Angina pectoris	783	146	152
Hip replacement	342	250	256
Knee replacement	344	373	367
Hip fracture	315	311	388
Kidney or urinary infection	396	449	526
Source: Ham *et al* (2003)			

- better procurement, including of medicines, where UK prices are the highest in Europe

- use of process improvements – for example, to reduce waiting times further and improve patient experience

- more investment in prevention, whether through reducing the prevalence of smoking, tackling childhood obesity or prescribing statins for people with certain heart conditions.

Most of these variations and facts have been known about for a long time. The challenging questions to ask are: Where to target? How much can be gained? How difficult is it going to be? and, above all, What will impel the necessary changes?

Potential areas of significant gain

Four areas have often been identified for significant productivity gain:

- **day-case activity** an important area for increasing productivity, with clear evidence of variation and known best practice

- **reductions in length of stay for common conditions** where current variation and known international practice suggest this is possible

- **reductions in avoidable admissions to hospital** where there is reasonably consistent medical opinion that there should in theory be no requirement for admission because the condition can be satisfactorily treated in primary care

- **improved management of chronic conditions** for example, to avoid emergency admissions through improved treatment compliance.

Day-case activity

As a recent analysis has shown (Farr 2006), the English national day-case rate for the 25 procedures originally identified by the Audit Commission stood at 67.2 per cent for the third quarter of 2005, compared with the target rate of 75 per cent. Actual rates between strategic health authority (SHA) areas varied from 73.6 per cent in South West London to 59.3 per cent in neighbouring in North West London.

The point here is not that such variations exist, but that they have persisted despite the Department of Health's long-term pressure for improvement. There has, in fact, been very little movement over the past five years, with rates creeping up at about 1 percentage point a year. Although some procedures are already at or above the target rate, others have further to go (*see* Figure 3 below). The suspicion is that, for whatever reason, the rates are more or less stuck, and have been for some time.

Reductions in length of stay

Around 30 health care resource groups (HRGs) account for 50 per cent of all elective inpatient episodes, and a similar number account for 50 per cent of all non-elective cases. Length of stay across hospitals within each of these HRGs varies significantly. Reducing those above the average to the current average might save about 4.8 million bed-days a year – perhaps about £1 billion at £200 per bed-day. A 10 per cent reduction across length of stay as a whole would save rather less – about 1 million bed-days. There will be good reason for at least some of the variation, and both the analysis and the savings figure are a little simplistic. Nevertheless, process improvements of the kind suggested by the Modernisation Agency and the new National NHS Innovation Institute ought to result in positive change.

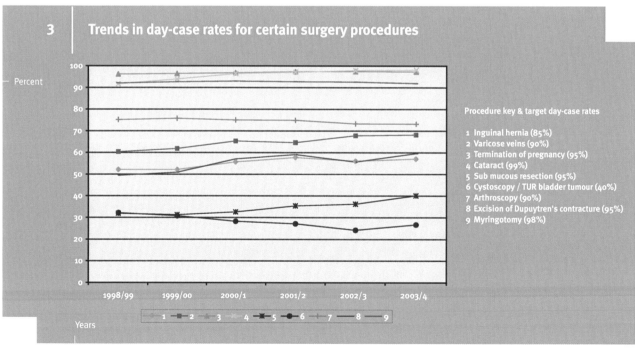

3 | **Trends in day-case rates for certain surgery procedures**

Procedure key & target day-case rates

1 Inguinal hernia (85%)
2 Varicose veins (90%)
3 Termination of pregnancy (95%)
4 Cataract (99%)
5 Sub mucous resection (95%)
6 Cystoscopy / TUR bladder tumour (40%)
7 Arthroscopy (90%)
8 Excision of Dupuytren's contracture (95%)
9 Myringotomy (98%)

Source: Audit Commission AHP

There are also international comparisons that can be used to demonstrate the possibilities. However, there are two cautionary points to bear in mind. First, as with day cases, there has been little apparent change in performance in the NHS over recent years – perhaps suggesting that achieving reductions in stay is harder than might be imagined.

Second, performance elsewhere in the world may not be so very different from that here. Table 2 below compares performance in England with that in Canada and Australia, both of which spend a little more than we do on health as a proportion of Gross Domestic Product (GDP) and have some similar features – for example, the use of a payment-by-results funding system. On this basis, Kaiser and perhaps elsewhere in the USA looks a distinct outlier. Making any international comparisons is fraught with difficulty and dangers. The point here is not to imply that achieving the kind of performance shown by some organisations in the US is impossible, but simply that the NHS is not alone in being unable to achieve it so far, although hospitals are expensive all over the world and budgets are generally under continual pressure. Furthermore, shorter lengths of stay may not always mean better care. It is also important to look at the costs and output overall, as well as those of individual institutions. Individual hospitals may be more efficient in the USA, but what matters is what we get in total for our money.

Avoidable admissions

Avoidable admissions – based on a range of 'ambulatory care-sensitive conditions' – account for about 15 per cent of all non-elective admissions, at an overall cost of just over £1 billion. In theory they should not happen, but in practice they do. Reducing variations in the numbers of these kinds of admissions would mean savings; reducing all avoidable admissions to zero would, in theory, generate the full £1 billion. However, primary care trusts (PCTs) and general practitioners would have to work extremely hard to achieve relatively small gains – a maximum of £3 million per PCT on the current numbers – not counting any costs that would be incurred by providing better primary care, and also assuming that trusts could realise the full amount of the cost reduction implied.

Chronic conditions

Better management of chronic conditions should yield dividends both in terms of patient health and in terms of efficiency, by reducing the number of hospital admissions – as Figure 4, p 69 shows when comparing actual against expected admissions – many of

2 | Comparison of average lengths of stay

Condition	England	Kaiser (USA)	Australia	Canada
Stroke	9.5	4.3	12.6	
Heart failure	5.3	3.7	11.1	7.0
Primary hip replacement	8.7	4.5	9.8	9.4
Primary knee replacement	8.3	4.2	7.7	10.4
Angina	2.8	2.2	5.1	
Source: Audit Commission/OECD 2006				

which are for chronic conditions. Shifting the overall curve *could* have big gains. And grounding 'frequent flyers' has become both a passion and an obsession for many in the NHS.

Results can be achieved – as Calderdale PCT has demonstrated by introducing eight community case managers and a number of other service changes, producing a reduction in admission rates as shown in Figure 4 opposite.

In Calderdale there are now about 25 fewer admissions per week compared with a year or so ago. The PCT estimates that its investment of about £500,000 has yielded significantly greater savings and improved care. There are examples elsewhere of good practice. But spreading such initiatives has always been a challenge, which so far has not been met successfully. The NHS also needs to increase its capacity to make accurate economic assessments of change both before and after the change, and to have the quality of data to match.

There are other potentially significant opportunities for improving productivity, either at the level of individual organisations, or across whole health communities. For example, expenditure on drugs represents a significant chunk of the total NHS spend, around 13 per cent, and costs have been rising faster than in other spending areas for many years. Prescribing has been subject to a panoply of policies, initiatives, data and advice aimed at achieving greater cost-effectiveness over a number of years. The single biggest efficiency gains in this area have been achieved by medicines coming off patent and national price deals. Prescribing neatly illustrates the point that it is clearly possible to improve productivity locally, but even with what look like a very good set of drivers to improve productivity, it is hard graft, and gains are often unspectacular.

Achieving productivity gains

Gordon Brown has focused recent microeconomic policies on what he describes as the 'five key drivers of productivity' – competition, enterprise, science and innovation, skills and investment. These elements are partly present in the NHS: the bones of a competitive market are being introduced for elective hospital care and may also develop in primary and community services. The introduction of private-sector providers has stimulated different approaches, and some NHS foundation trust chief executives are claiming a greater entrepreneurial attitude. Some general practitioners and secondary-care clinicians have always been regarded as entrepreneurial.

New technologies have often been a double-edged sword – with the NHS concerned as much about cost increases as about the new possibilities that they open up. But the great white hope is clearly the National Programme for Information Technology (IT). Although it has not moved as fast as originally desired, once it is implemented and accepted it can still offer the potential for radical improvement. There has also been more emphasis on changing the skill mix and improving the skills of different groups of staff through, for example, prescribing changes and backing this approach with a more flexible pay system. One PCT Chief Executive has quietly boasted that his out-of-hours service is now nurse-led and is operating more cheaply and more efficiently than the GP-led service of his neighbour, with whom he is about to merge. However, wider evidence to support such

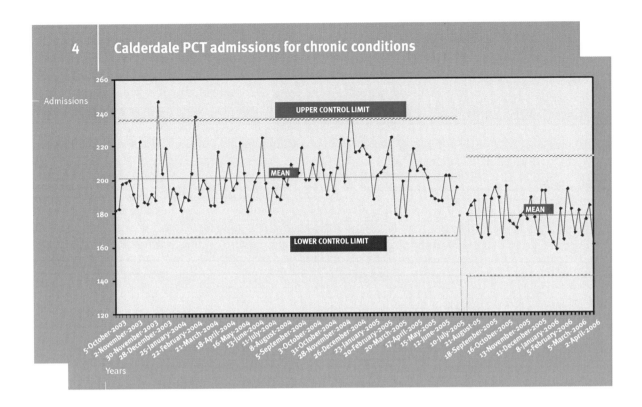

4 | Calderdale PCT admissions for chronic conditions

anecdotal claims is in short supply. Even if there were such evidence, questions remain as to whether the NHS has the managerial capacity and clinician support to take advantage of these opportunities.

Finally, there is no doubt that the NHS has had significant investment in both revenue and capital. This in itself has probably served temporarily to reduce headline productivity growth as it has in other industries, given lags between changes in inputs and changes in outputs. The question is whether the NHS can now capitalise on its investment as others do.

For that to happen, the following steps will be necessary.

First, there needs to be greater clarity as to what drivers can be used in the new world of NHS system reform and what effect they will have. Providers will be heavily influenced through the financing system, which can seek to achieve greater efficiency. Provider quality improvements are more likely to be addressed through contracts (the national tariff means that local pricing for greater efficiency is not possible), by competition in elective care through patient choice, and also potentially by external performance assessment ('star ratings'). Purchasers will be driven in part by financial incentives but probably more by targets, performance management and any rating system. Their aim should be to maximise overall outputs, not just those related to secondary care, for the money allocated to them.

There also needs to be clarity about objectives. It is not wholly clear, for example, whether substantial additional hospital activity will be required – unlike in 2000, when it was assumed (incorrectly, as it has turned out) that very significant increases would be required in order to reduce waiting times, with money being provided and plans laid accordingly. International comparisons suggest that some increase in intervention rates will be needed, although the picture varies. However, within the NHS there is no clear link between resources, need and admissions – PCTs below weighted-capitation target levels of funding do not appear to have fewer admissions than expected, given the established need – roughly as many are above the line of best fit as are below it. Conversely, those above target funding do not necessarily seem to provide more output than expected. This is true of total admissions as well as for a number of specific disease conditions.

This point is important, because a hospital's response to financial pressure may be to try and increase income. This may help headline productivity figures but will not achieve wider objectives. It is also important in setting expectations, aligning incentives and measuring what happens. If the goal were simply to increase hospital activity, setting PCTs' cost-weighted activity targets appropriately – as was done with some success in the 1990s – would provide the right incentive. But such tactics attracted criticism then, with arguments that the incentive produced perverse and undesirable outcomes.

Second, the financing system and the way trusts and PCTs react to it will clearly be critical. It contains powerful incentives and should, in theory, drive positive changes – for example, in length of stay and staff utilisation. The way it works in practice, however, needs careful and continuous evaluation. In 2004/5 there was something of a controlled experiment between foundation trusts on the one hand, operating under Payment by Results, and NHS trusts on the other, operating under the 'old' financial regime. Experience was mixed and at best inconclusive. Surprisingly perhaps, elective activity fell slightly in both sets of trusts, but emergency activity grew less strongly in the foundation sector. There were some signs that foundation trusts marginally improved their length of stay whereas it worsened in other acute trusts (*see* Figure 5 opposite).

However, foundation trusts increased their income by 13 per cent and their expenditure by 14 per cent, compared with 10.7 per cent and 11.4 per cent in NHS trusts. At the end of the year, there was little difference in the change in reference costs between the two sectors (*see* Figure 6 opposite).

The most that can be said is that it is early days yet – and also perhaps that, not surprisingly, large hospitals are not as fleet of foot in responding to financial incentives as are GP practices. The impact of patient choice has yet to be really felt, although some argue that the early London choice pilots showed potentially promising results.

Third, a savings target of 2.7 per cent has been included in the tariff for 2006/7, and doubtless further targets will be included in the future; but there is more that could be done. It should be possible to have a more aggressive policy for some HRGs beyond encouraging further take-up of the current basket of day-case procedures through tariff setting. The Department should review potential areas for improvement with clinicians, drawing on, for example, experience in the USA but also elsewhere, and set tariff prices according to the productivity outcome desired – essentially for much shorter lengths of stay. It should declare the approach and the possible outcome some two years in advance of the change, so signalling the intention and giving time for adjustment. And just as the Modernisation Agency had successful programmes that underpinned access targets for elective care and in Accident and Emergency, so its successor should be commissioned to support the changes implied by the tariff. This might be a rolling programme.

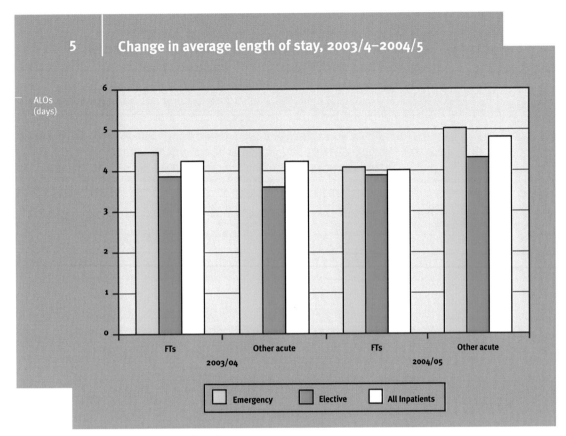

5 | Change in average length of stay, 2003/4–2004/5

ALOs (days)

FTs   Other acute   FTs   Other acute

2003/04   2004/05

Emergency   Elective   All Inpatients

Source: Audit Commission (2005)

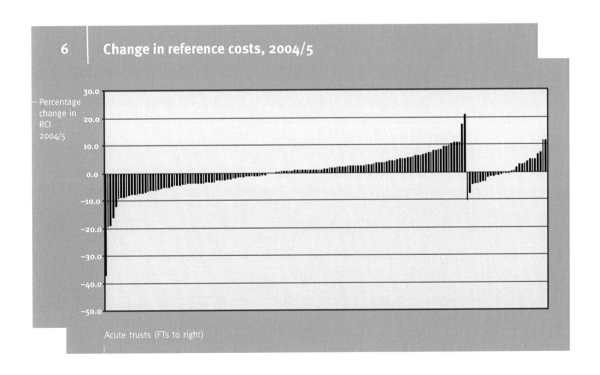

6 | Change in reference costs, 2004/5

Percentage change in RCI 2004/5

Acute trusts (FTs to right)

Fourth, quality improvement and associated productivity gains in hospitals need better measurement and better incentives. The measurement would come from instituting a more consistent and rigorous programme, based perhaps on generic health status measures such as, perhaps, the Short-form 36 (SF36). The incentives would come from identifying the performance – in health outcome terms – of individual units within trusts, and external assessment and publication of their performance in ratings that would in turn provide greater public accountability and inform choice. The data might also be used to begin genuine payment by *results* rather than payment by activity. This would also provide a much clearer and objective framework for testing performance in individual units, potentially opening the way to specific licensing or franchising.

None of this would happen overnight, and there are clear dangers in trying to run before mastering walking – particularly with the tariff. However, it would be important now to set out a clear and coherent programme along these lines and work towards it.

Turning to PCTs, targets need to be set that combine efficiency with health gain and that more clearly link expenditure and outputs (or even outcomes). An efficiency target alone is unlikely to capture the imaginations of the PCT and their clinicians. Few targets have linked efficiency and health gain, the main exception perhaps being the reduction in emergency bed-days. Such targets may be hard to come by nationally, although 'avoidable admissions' might be a potential area. If this is the case, it would be more appropriate to agree health and efficiency targets with individual PCTs based on their own profiles and with clinical involvement.

The performance management and assessment system would then need to be geared to match. This would not mean abrogating national targets or policies – it would still be possible to have a common set of NHS standards (for example, for waiting times). Such an approach would, however, also speak more clearly to potential joint commissioning between health and local government. In the longer term it should be possible to go on to combine measures of PCT performance based on programme budget data and outputs or outcomes for disease categories, linked perhaps to national service frameworks. This would bring together performance and productivity in primary as well as secondary care and acknowledge the role that an effective local prevention strategy might have.

In addition, more attention needs to be given to the capacity and capability of PCTs and, with that, the development and operation of practice-based commissioning on which many hopes rest for better demand management and improved efficiency. The Fitness for Purpose assessments planned for each PCT are obvious starting points for the former, but need to be supplemented with a stronger analytical and economic capability. The outcome of the assessment process should also be directly linked to PCT commissioning plans and potentially to individually agreed targets, as set out above. There would then be a more objective basis for determining progress and whether specific functions might need to be supported or addressed more radically – perhaps through outsourcing, which is only possible if there is clear specification and clear measurement, neither of which seem to be present currently.

Practice-based commissioning should help once it becomes effective. However, GP fundholding and successor developments such as Total Purchasing Pilots were variable in their achievement and bite. Practice-based commissioning needs rigorous implementation locally against a clearly defined set of outcome criteria and local incentive structures aligned with local (or national) targets.

Finally, the further crucial element in prompting higher productivity is likely to be simply that less cash may be available for the service. Tight funding has been associated with greater efficiency (as for example in the 1990s). Of all the essential steps, this seems to be the most guaranteed.

References

Farr M (2006). 'Databriefing'. *Health Service Journal*, vol 116 (5999), p 21.

Ham C, York N, Sutch S, Shaw R (2003). 'Hospital bed utilisation in the NHS, Kaiser Permanente, and the US Medicare programme: analysis of routine data'. *British Medical Journal*, vol 327, p 1257.

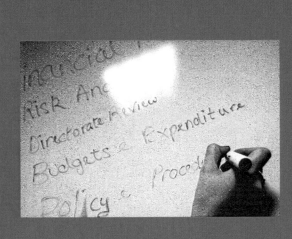

Part 3

Managing a low-growth future

Key questions

- What would a significant step-down in funding mean in political terms and for the ability of the NHS to meet future targets?
- How would trusts manage this reduction, given cost pressures, and still implement ongoing policies such as Payment by Results and patient choice?
- What are the prospects for successfully controlling spending and eradicating deficits?

Targets, targets, targets
Prospects for successful implementation of current NHS reforms

Mike Farrar

Targets, targets, targets
Prospects for successful implementation of current NHS reforms

Mike Farrar

Introduction

These are difficult times to be an National Health Service (NHS) manager. To believe some of the current news coverage would be to believe that the NHS is on the verge of collapse, with massive redundancies, spiralling costs, and multitudes of bureaucrats robbing frontline services of much-needed cash. However, to believe other commentaries offered on the problems would be to accept that all of the current issues were predictable and are a facet of the reform programme biting, and that ultimately this pain is necessary to achieve a radically different but more productive health service. For the casual observer of the NHS, this debate might appear to be rather esoteric, despite its current political importance. But understanding what is happening in the NHS now is essential for those of us charged with implementing change and delivering the current NHS reforms and targets within the resources available.

NHS managers currently need to 'think more and do less'. We desperately need to look more intelligently at the implementation of the reforms, at the nature of the financial challenge we face (both its cause and its effects), and at the impact that both might have on the ability of the NHS to continue to hit its key targets. Overall, there is a need to examine and understand the complex relationship between the expectations that the government has set for the service (through the targets it has set and the resources it has made available), the prospects for their achievement within budget, and the contribution, for good or ill, that the aspiration to reform the way in which the NHS functions will make to this.

The modernisation or reform agenda is in itself perceived to be a complex one. Many NHS leaders and clinicians reportedly find it difficult to piece together coherently. Yet at its heart, it is relatively simple. The reform of the NHS is the transformation from a top-down, centrally driven service to one where the local dynamics between competing providers and intelligent, discerning commissioners (exploiting the new choice of provider available to them and the population they serve) lead to sustainable quality improvement and increased value for the taxpayers' money. In summary, it is a transformation whereby the government's demands of the service are replaced by the public's demands as customers, increasing the desire of providers to meet customer demand, and so driving up quality and value for money.

These dynamics fundamentally change the incentives within the NHS and will – in theory – provide the platform for achieving and then exceeding the NHS Plan targets set back in 2000. They also serve to incentivise greater efficiency, greater productivity and lower costs, thereby ensuring that the NHS can live within its means – particularly once NHS spending achieves the level of the European Union (EU) average and the current record levels of investment settle down to more modest levels of growth.

Despite the logic of the policy (and indeed there appears to be little disagreement between the major political parties on this direction of travel), there is concern that there has been little reform in practice and that most achievement of the milestones towards the 2008 NHS Plan targets has come about through supply-side growth (increases in the numbers of doctors, nurses and beds), with increases rather than reductions in unit cost and therefore little demonstrable productivity gain. Indeed, as the end-of-year accounts are prepared for 2005/6, the financial position of the NHS is of even greater concern, and for some commentators the question is one of the price of reform, and whether the NHS will be able to afford to hit its targets at all.

The real issue, however, is about the costs of *not* reforming. The current financial problems relate not to change in the way the NHS operates but to the lack of change.

Pressures to reform

At its simplest, the experience of the NHS to date can be captured in the following equations:

Financial health + targets	=	short-term supply-side growth + inefficiency
Financial health – targets	=	variable NHS performance + inefficiency
Financial pressure – targets	=	unfocused rationalisation + service cuts + increases in waiting lists and times
Financial pressure + targets	=	reform + productivity + efficiency

While these represent sweeping generalisations about the nature of NHS performance, it is possible to attribute these characteristics to different phases of the history of the NHS over the past 20 years.

While the most recent three or four years can in general be characterised by high levels of supply-side growth but with little attention paid to productivity and efficiency, the next phase the NHS is about to enter will be different – at the very least, out of necessity. The NHS has challenging targets to meet by 2008, by which time it is committed to a maximum journey time of 18 weeks from referral to a bed in hospital for all specialties. But there are current financial problems to contend with, and the likely level of future funding growth will halve after the next spending review.

In this case, the financial pressure plus the targets should be a spur for greater modernisation. Necessity becomes the mother of invention, and reform not the catalyst for further financial pressure, but the solution to it. The next phase will increase the pace of reform, particularly in the drive for greater productivity and efficiency on the provider side.

Hitting the targets through reform

So what evidence is there to support a belief that the NHS will hit all its targets within the resources available, and that this will have been aided and abetted by reform rather than hindered by it?

First, it is worth noting that there appears to be little or no correlation between financial balance, evidence of reform (as measured by the number of foundation trusts and therefore the full introduction of Payment by Results) and utilisation of secondary care. Indeed, South Yorkshire and Northumberland Tyne and Wear, both in the top five strategic health authorities (SHAs) when rated on finances and reform, appear to have the highest level of hospital utilisation. South Yorkshire – ironically the first health system in the country to have all its acute hospitals with foundation trust status – also enjoys the highest number of hospital beds per head of population. It is certainly not possible to find any causal link between an inability to hit targets and the introduction of reforms, or a link between introduction of reforms and poor financial performance.

So what does lie behind the successful implementation of reform, maintaining financial balance and any prediction of future achievement of targets?

Good management ...

The answer, I would suggest, is that implementation of health policy and achievement of targets, like the financial performance of the NHS, has been and remains predominantly psychological rather than technical. The NHS functions and, it can be argued, relatively effectively, on the quality of its leadership and the expertise and commitment of its staff. Sadly, it lacks the intelligent information, the streamlined processes, and the comprehensive systematising of best practice to enable it to exploit its human capability to the full. Indeed, it is the lack of such organisational infrastructure that makes it necessary for the NHS to place its activities onto a more commercial, customer-orientated footing. Once again the drivers for this change emanate from the current reform programme.

... but a need for 'intelligent' information ...

The reform programme will generate a much more effective 'corporate dashboard' that will allow the NHS to understand its business better, pinpoint problems, identify success, allow it to spread best practice, predict failure and intervene where necessary. Already NHS organisations are using benchmarking data to understand their productivity gains. West Yorkshire organisations, for example, all know their share of the £21m worth of savings from reducing unnecessary follow-ups, from the 19,000 inpatients who could be treated as day cases, and from the huge savings to be made by routinely admitting on the day of surgery.

Recently, diagnostic work by the foundation trust enabled all three major NHS trusts in West Yorkshire SHA to determine that compulsory redeployment would enable major workforce reductions without the need for redundancies as they right-sized their respective workforces. The world of the NHS organisation is changing rapidly, and the financial pressure coupled with the impending targets are speeding this transformation.

... and demand management ...

The second area of evidence relates to the recent history of West Yorkshire SHA. West Yorkshire has assessed the cost of achieving the milestones towards the 2008 access targets and predicted their cost (assuming no effective increase in the management of demand). The figures are revealing.

Costings in Figure 1 below are based on the increased cost of secondary activity for main surgical specialties, using the average speciality tariff and weighted-average health resource group (HRG) standard-stay tariff with a 7.3 per cent market forces factor (MFF) uplift.

Figures for 2007/8 and 2008/9 assume that all the progress towards the target of 18 weeks is based on purchasing extra hospital activity, with no contribution from any reduction in demand. Even at these levels, they would be affordable within primary care trust (PCT) growth; but it is known that PCTs have had some success in the past with management of demand (in advance of the introduction of practice-based commissioning). Between 2002/3 and 2004/5, for example, West Yorkshire PCTs reduced demand in GP referrals by 5.6 per cent and elective activity by 1 per cent – although performance was massively variable between the 15 organisations (–16 per cent GP referrals in South and West Bradford to +5 per cent GP referrals in South Huddersfield, for example). This is why the additional actual secondary-care expenditure in the corresponding years is below the £10 million mark.

Here again, with the advent of better commissioning through new PCTs and the introduction of practice-based commissioning, it can be argued that the reform programme will be a positive force in enabling NHS targets to be achieved within the resources available.

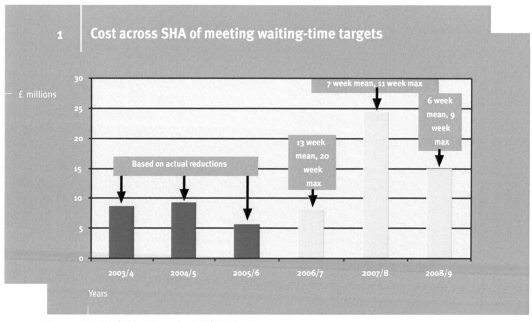

Source: West Yorkshire Strategic Health Authority

... and careful capacity planning ...

One of the risks of the reform programme, however, is the variety of assumptions that are being made by providers and commissioners about the capacity required to deal with non-elective care. At present in West Yorkshire – a trend probably reflected in many places – trusts are forecasting a 0.2 per cent increase in non-elective activity and a 2.43 per cent increase in elective activity. The backdrop to this is a 0.27 per cent increase in the population and a 4.6 per cent increase in funding per capita (net of cost inflation). While this again looks affordable within PCT budgets, the significant aspect is that commissioners agree with the assumptions that trusts are making on elective growth but are planning on a 1 per cent *drop* in non-elective activity, representing a 6 per cent difference in expected activity by 2009/10.

The issue here is the costs to the commissioners if trust assumptions are borne out, or alternatively, the costs to the providers of maintaining under-utilised capacity should commissioner assumptions be borne out. In this circumstance, there could be unforeseen consequences of the reforms, such as intervention in the marketplace by the strategic bodies (or regulators), supply-induced demand, or major contract disputes, bringing with them their own potential costs.

Conclusion

It is essential that all NHS organisations, at all levels, look carefully at why the NHS has incurred significant financial problems. This examination should not just be a technical accounting exercise, but should look for psychological explanations too.

Good behaviours, good information, good leadership are vital. In time, the corporate dashboard of the NHS will enable a greater application of technology to the management of resource, but in the short term the changes to the incentives facing managers and clinicians will generate better practice, higher quality and efficiency. Are the NHS targets still affordable? Yes, clearly; even if the costs of the extra secondary-care activity were borne by PCTs as they currently operate, there is sufficient growth in most parts of the country to enable them to manage, and the strategic reserve powers for new SHAs will serve to smooth out the variations in performance and purchasing power in the short term. But more to the point, the NHS will respond to the reform agenda. Trusts will seek greater efficiencies. The focus on workforce will intensify in a move to 'right-size' acute capacity, and the incentives to manage demand will settle in and grow.

Money is tight, but the NHS is still enjoying record levels of growth, and the taxpayer has a right to see a more productive, more efficient, better-governed and higher-quality service in return. The NHS will deliver.

Participants

Professor John Appleby	Chief Economist, King's Fund
Sir Roger Bannister	Leeds Castle Foundation Trustee
Dame Carol Black	President, Royal College of Physicians
Professor Nick Bosanquet	Honorary Fellow, Imperial College of Science, Technology and Medicine
Sir Cyril Chantler	Chairman, King's Fund
Anita Charlesworth	Director, Public Services HM Treasury
Dr Will Cavendish	Director of Strategy, Department of Health
Robert Chote	Director, The Institute for Fiscal Studies
Caroline Clarke	Finance Director, Homerton University Hospital Trust
Baroness Cumberlege	Senior Associate, King's Fund; Leeds Castle Foundation Trustee
Niall Dickson	Chief Executive, King's Fund
Dr Jennifer Dixon	Director of Policy, King's Fund
Professor Nancy Devlin	Senior Associate, King's Fund; Professor of Health Economics, City University
Richard Douglas	Director of Finance and Investment, Department of Health
Nigel Edwards	Director of Policy, NHS Confederation
Mike Farrar	Chief Executive, West Yorkshire Strategic Health Authority
Dr Julien Forder	Project Lead for the Wanless Social Care Review; Deputy Director, PSSRU, London School of Economics
Jeremy Hurst	Head of Health Policy Unit, Organisation for Economic Co-operation and Development

Professor Julian Le Grand   Richard Titmuss Professor of Social Policy, London
                                 School of Economics

Professor Alan Maynard   Professor of Health Economics, University of York

Andy McKeon   Managing Director of Health, Audit Commission

Professor Carol Propper   Director, CMPO, University of Bristol

Jonathan Slater   Director of Health, Prime Minister's Delivery Unit

Simon Stevens   President, United Health Group

Alison Tonge   Director of Finance and Estates, Stockport PCT